SMART MEDICINE

SMART
MEDICINE

HOW THE CHANGING ROLE
OF DOCTORS WILL
REVOLUTIONIZE HEALTH CARE

WILLIAM HANSON, M.D.

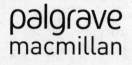

First published in 2011 by
PALGRAVE MACMILLAN®
in the United States—a division of St. Martin's Press LLC,
175 Fifth Avenue, New York, NY 10010.

Where this book is distributed in the UK, Europe and the rest of the world,
this is by Palgrave Macmillan, a division of Macmillan Publishers Limited,
registered in England, company number 785998, of Houndmills,
Basingstoke, Hampshire RG21 6XS.

Palgrave Macmillan is the global academic imprint of the above companies
and has companies and representatives throughout the world.

Palgrave® and Macmillan® are registered trademarks in the United States, the
United Kingdom, Europe and other countries.

ISBN-13: 978-0-230-62115-2

Library of Congress Cataloging-in-Publication Data

Hanson, William, M.D.
    Smart medicine : how the changing role of doctors will revolutionize
health care / William Hanson, M.D.
        p. cm.
    Includes bibliographical references and index.
    ISBN 978-0-230-62115-2 (hardback)
    1. Medical innovations. I. Title.

RA418.5.M4H36 2011
610.285—dc22   2010049047

A catalogue record of the book is available from the British Library.

Design by Newgen Imaging Systems (P) Ltd., Chennai, India.

First edition: June 2011

10 9 8 7 6 5 4 3 2 1

Printed in the United States of America.

CONTENTS

Part IV   New Models of Care

ACKNOWLEDGMENTS

This book represents the second in a series on the future of medicine, a topic that's increasingly relevant as the present recedes ever more rapidly into the rearview mirror, one that was originally suggested by Airié Stuart, senior vice president and publisher, and Luba Ostashevsky, my editor, at Palgrave Macmillan. My agent Eric Lupfer, at William Morris Endeavor, has been an invaluable counselor through the course of both books.

Many friends have contributed in one way or another to various aspects of *Smart Medicine*, including Peter and Eileen Quinn, Bill and Marge Schwab and Hugh and Carolyn Braithwaite who helped me kicked around various titles. PJ Brennan helped with a reality check on some of the material, as did Susan Philips. I am also very fortunate to work in a department, hospital, health system and university where I am surrounded by talented and competent colleagues and role models, some of whom appear in the pages of the book. I'd like to have been able to include and identify all of them.

One of my oldest friends and earliest mentors, Howard Steel, did a word-by-word read-through of the manuscript and brought his inimitable style and grace to the process of improving the work. Meg Davis helped once again—this time with feedback about the book's design.

The biggest thanks belong to my wife, Beth, and my children, Addison, Watson and Callaghan, who've been a source of inspiration and feedback for every word—and patiently kept checking on my progress as I wrote right up to the deadline. My siblings, Ellen, Beth, John and Chris have each helped in their own way, as has my mother, Ann. My father remains my most important role model and the kind of doctor I think we're all looking for: insightful, compassionate and responsible, he was a physician for all seasons.

DISCLAIMER

Except where so referenced, the medical cases in this book do not refer to individuals but are composites used to illustrate a wide range of diagnoses, treatments, risks and benefits associated with a variety of medical technologies and situations. Names and characteristics are used fictitiously. Resemblance to any real person is unintended and entirely coincidental.

INTRODUCTION

S*mart Medicine,* like my previous book *The Edge of Medicine,* is designed to be a look at the health field during an era of rapid and, some might say, chaotic change. Money that once flowed limitlessly into medical research and care has unquestionably begun to dry up. At the same time, new technologies with seemingly limitless promise, like genomics and stem cell therapy, are poised to enter the arena.

As with many healthy industries, medicine is constantly in ferment. Expansive forces generate new treatments and tools, as well as the specialists and specialties that deliver them. Then limitations focus the application of the resulting new disciplines and cull out older ones that are no longer competitive.

Like banking, manufacturing and publishing, medicine is finally automating—albeit later. The relationship between the provider of the service and the consumer will be radically remade in the process, as it has been with each of the other industries. The consumer will have much more in the way of choice, autonomy and leverage in the consumption of medical care, and the industry will become much more nimble as a result.

Finally, medical providers and care models are changing, too. The medical trainee was once an apprentice—indentured to her profession for a term of what has traditionally been quite hard labor. Unlike almost every other professional career, medicine has traditionally required its trainees to put family rearing, the elimination of educational debt and the accrual of a nest egg on hold for a decade or more. And, until recently, the culture of medicine was all-consuming—one in which doctors often placed the needs of their patients before those of their own families. But as medicine has increasingly become a crisis-oriented, round-the-clock juggernaut, and as studies have shown a correlation between provider fatigue and patient care errors, new models of care have developed. The heroic, indefatigable, fearless and flawless physician once portrayed on television and in movies has given way to more realistic depictions of doctors with lives outside of medicine, who sometimes make mistakes. There's a new emphasis on team-based care, both in Hollywood depictions of the profession and in the real world.

In the first section of the book, we'll explore what modern medicine looks like—the people who are entering the field and the way they'll be trained. The second section will look to the past—to previous periods of enormous change in medicine and the forces that shaped it during its evolution. In the third section, we'll see how the computerization of medicine will allow us to provide smarter, safer and more efficient care, while in the fourth, and last section, I'll illustrate some of the solutions that are evolving in response to medicine's flaws, the threats they represent to the complacent and the promise they may provide for patients in the future.

PART I

MODERN MEDICINE

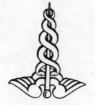

The modern hospital is a fast-paced world of almost limitless promise. Patients arrive through the front door and the emergency ward, in ambulances and helicopters. They leave on crutches, in wheelchairs and in hearses. Human organs fly through the night in coolers to be transplanted into recipients hundreds of miles away. To some, no illness seems insurmountable. Yet death always prevails in the end. One could argue that we've forgotten how to die gracefully and peacefully.

In this first part of the book, we'll see what health care looks like today. We'll meet the young people who are entering the profession as students—those who will lead us into the future using new and better techniques and methods of communication. We'll visit medical school classrooms of the future and listen to some of the timeless lessons of the past—the ones that have endured through centuries of relentless change.

CHAPTER 1

BED NINE DID DIE

Like many of today's doctors, I no longer carry a pager. I use my smartphone for all personal and professional communications. This has the benefit of consolidating a variety of functions onto a single device and means that I have less weight to carry on my hip. I spend parts of many days wearing scrubs, and the scrub-pant drawstring is less sturdy than a belt as a platform for waist-based devices. Interns and residents who may have to carry a hospital phone, their own phone and a code-red beeper often develop an unsightly sag in the scrubs where the pants pull down. During a my residency, when I needed to carry both a pager and one of the original, heavy cell phones, I briefly considered wearing a fanny pack or one of those utility belts worn by police or army officers but quickly decided that it just wouldn't look right on me. Of course, the downside to using my cell phone as the single point of contact is that, as a physician, I can't afford to screen calls because a lot of people I don't know need to be able to contact me for medical emergencies. So I get a lot of chaff along with the wheat when I answer unfamiliar numbers.

My smartphone displays a high-tech white analog clock face on a black background when I plug it in to recharge. This virtual timepiece can be configured to act as an alarm clock, too. One night it dawned on me that I could actually do away with my old electric alarm, which I'd laboriously reset after every power outage, and instead use the phone's clock for that function. After some fiddling, I selected a ringtone labeled "Inspired Asian Morning" as my wake-up reveille. It features some double-reeded instrument, like an Eastern variant of the oboe, playing a rising, quavering note against a backdrop of drums. I like this because it wakes me more gently than the old alarm clock did and doesn't bother my wife if I need to wake up earlier than she does.

After some use, I've found that this wedding of smartphone with alarm clock is convenient and saves bedside space; but, as with many marriages, it comes with pros and cons. Once I dismiss the alarm, the "You've got mail" prompt automatically pops up. And I can't always resist the urge to see what rolled in during the night. Occasionally I find a message from a friend in a different time zone; sometimes there's nothing but a few stray spams. In reality, there's almost never anything important enough to warrant postponing a good toothbrushing, but it's become an almost Pavlovian response: the alarm sounds and, like a well-trained dog, I open my email.

One recent morning I awakened to find a message that had arrived earlier, at 3:02 AM, entitled "Attending Mortality Form Notification." The sending party was someone, or perhaps some thing, called "Death Forms Application." Neither the subject nor the sender fell into any category I recognized immediately, and both sounded vaguely ominous. So I further postponed the dental hygiene and after some investigation found that I had also gotten a text message at 2:50 AM, about 15 minutes earlier, one that hadn't awakened me. After checking my phone log (and further waking from my groggy condition), I remembered that I had gotten and answered a couple of calls from the hospital shortly before midnight.

This probably warrants a quick bit of personal disclosure. Like some of you, I have my own individual, multi-tiered response to cell-phone-based communications. As it happens, not through any particular design, my alerts all have an Eastern flavor. The "Inspired Asian Morning" alarm clock harmonizes nicely with my phone's "Chi Gong" ringtone, which sounds like one of those giant hanging gongs used in Asian temples. I prefer *my* alerts to some of the alternatives I hear around the hospital: the opening bars of "A Hard Day's Night" or the howling of a submarine "Dive!" I've come to believe that you can tell a lot about a person by the alerts they choose, and it's no surprise that an entire industry has grown up around ringtones.

I have chosen not to get any notification about new emails. A colleague set his phone set to vibrate with every new mail message—checking his email became a visible, twitchy habit. His wife thought he had developed a tic and forced him to buy a phone that couldn't be configured to notify him about new emails. I prefer to check mine every now and then to see if anything new has arrived. Recent neurological research has actually shown that these random email alerts trigger little surges of neurotransmitters in the brain, simultaneously signaling stress and pleasure…like little dominatrices.

My incoming text messages are configured to sound a single "Light Chime," also Asian in flavor. And both my phone and text message alerts are set to vibrate simultaneously with the audio alert so I don't miss a medical emergency when, for example, as is often the case, two or more of my children are in a heated discussion about some piece of disputed property, like the shotgun position in the car, or food. This seemingly redundant pairing of vibrate and sound is actually designed to act as a "belt and suspenders": vibration notifies me when it's too loud to hear, and sound does so when I'm already vibrating as I when drive in my bouncy Jeep.

On the morning at issue, I had actually gotten three different types of electronic messages during the night. One of them, the phone call, had awakened me, and two of them, the email and text messages, hadn't. I actually smiled to myself because this alerting configuration that I'd carefully customized had worked exactly as I intended: I *did* want to be awakened by phone calls but *not* by texts or emails.

As I lay there that morning in the pre-dawn dark, it occurred to me that my father, who was a general internist, also had mornings like this, when he awakened bleary after a night interrupted by patient-related phone calls. But he never carried a cell phone, never got the hang of email and certainly never texted. The type of medicine I practice is definitely not my father's medicine.

I had been covering the intensive care service that week, which meant that I got a lot of calls every night. These calls were related to bed management in our crowded ICU (intensive care unit) as well as questions from the residents who were in-house, dealing with the issues that crop up with regularity during any given night. We also "round"—visiting each patient's bedside several times each day—because critically ill patients change continually in one direction or another, and their care requires lots of round-the-clock fine tuning.

Margarita Latincic was one of my patients that week. I met her on rounds after surgery for a collection of pus in her belly, although she was still sedated and on a respirator at the time.

She was 69 years old and had been admitted to the hospital several times for the same problem over the past two months. Mrs. Latincic had initially developed inflammation and infection around her colon months earlier as a result of a condition called *diverticulitis*, in which little pockets develop in the wall of the large bowel. Diverticular disease is usually asymptomatic but can result in bleeding into the bowel, known as *diverticulosis*, or in an infection. Hoping to avoid a big operation, her doctors had initially drained a large collection of pus around the bowel via a catheter inserted through the skin by radiologists, but that had only worked briefly, and she went on to be readmitted for dehydration and kidney failure. Eventually, after several admissions, it became obvious that open surgery was needed to remove the infected bowel. This was her third major surgery, and there was concern about whether her system could take the stress.

Years earlier, Mrs. Latincic had developed an unusual liver disease called *primary biliary cirrhosis* in which the bile ducts become inflamed, probably as some sort of autoimmune reaction. As is often the case, the problem eventually progressed to the point that she required a liver transplant. Her first replacement liver lasted for about ten years and then failed. She then underwent a second, inevitably more complicated, liver transplant along with a simultaneous kidney transplant from the same donor.

The issue of retransplantation comes up often in ethical debates. With the scarcity of available organs and long waiting lists, ethicists ask if each potential recipient should be treated equally regardless of prior transplantation history, or should patients who've already been transplanted once rank lower in priority than first-time recipients. I know of one patient, a rabbi, who has received three livers over the course of several years.

Successful transplants can result in significant improvements in the lives of recipients. A patient who had been bedbound on oxygen prior to lung transplantation can return to breathing normally. An avid tennis player I know returned to the court after his heart transplant. The same is true for liver and kidney patients like Mrs. Latincic.

But this good comes with a cost. Almost every transplanted patient spends the rest of his life on drugs that suppress the immune system, and the immune system's role is to stave off infections and cancer. Immunosuppressed patients are at significantly increased risk from bacteria, from their own cells that "go rogue" and become malignant, as well as from immune cells that come along with the transplanted organ. In graft-versus-host disease, the transplanted organ's cells essentially attack the recipient.

Mrs. Latincic came to the ICU after an operation in which the inflamed section of her bowel was removed and the colon was then sewn back together. At first, everything appeared to be fine, although she was still on a ventilator and I noted that her heart rate was higher than normal after this kind of surgery. She was also hyperventilating and her kidneys weren't putting out enough urine. I wasn't surprised by the latter because I anticipated that she would need a little more intravenous (IV) fluid to replace the blood and serum lost during the operation. Also, for 24 to 28 hours after a big operation, fluid leaks out of the blood vessels into the tissues as part of a general inflammatory reaction, like a total body bruise; these patients appear to be dehydrated even though they may end up weighing more than they did before the operation when they started getting their needed transfusions.

During morning rounds that first day, I told the team to give her a liter or two of intravenous saline to see if her heart rate would come down. I also asked them to see if she was able to breathe on her own. In order to be safely taken off the ventilator after an operation, the patient must be awake and strong, and the lungs must be working. When I came back later in the day, she had gotten several more liters of IV fluid but still wasn't urinating enough. Also, her heart rate was still well over 100, which is high. She was awake enough to wince and point at her stomach, over the area of the surgery, indicating that it hurt. While the belly pain was normal, the whole constellation of other issues suggested that all was not well, and we decided to keep her on the ventilator overnight, which turned out to be a good thing.

Medicine is usually described as both a *science* and an *art*. The decision to keep this patient on the ventilator that afternoon falls on the art side of the equation. By all objective respiratory criteria at that point, Mrs. Latincic was ready to breathe on her own, but the high heart rate and low urine output were analogous to the cracking of twigs to an army sentry. They suggested that something was looming out there and that we should be extra vigilant.

Over the next 48 hours, Mrs. Latincic's situation gradually worsened. Her heart rate remained high and her blood pressure began to drop. Her kidneys stopped making urine altogether. She also developed a fever, and her lungs began to fill up with fluid so that she required more and more oxygen through the ventilator. She was developing the group of problems known as *sepsis* (a general inflammatory reaction throughout the body) and *adult respiratory distress syndrome*, wherein the lungs become "leaky."

At this point we engaged some help from several different special-ist teams. *Transplant infectious disease* is a sub-sub-specialty of plain old infectious disease, which is in turn a sub-specialty of internal medicine, one of medicine's traditional core specialties. These super-specialists are typi-cally only found at a transplant center like ours. We also contacted the renal team—the nephrologists—because it began to look like she'd need to start on dialysis as her kidneys failed.

Mrs. Latincic's core family members included her husband and two sons. They were very experienced with intensive care units, having witnessed her two prior transplants and the more recent hospitalizations for diverticulitis. Like many families, they spent a lot of time watching the monitors as they sat at her bedside. We briefed them frequently, but they were well aware that things were not proceeding in the right direction just from watching her vital signs and the expressions on the caregivers' faces.

The two sons sat vigil by the bedside. Their father had been there imme-diately after surgery, when things seemed straightforward, but was strangely absent as her course deteriorated. When we asked the sons whether he would be available to sign a consent form for interventions like dialysis, the older one explained that they shared power of attorney and could speak for their mother legally. Usually this role would fall to a spouse, but Mr. Latincic had, as they put it, "lost his mind" the last time she was critically ill. And the sons explained that this time he was staying at home but was extremely upset and felt we, the care team of doctors and nurses, were killing her. They also indicated that he had a gun.

In a previous era, we might have dismissed this information as interest-ing but not really relevant—but not anymore. On September 17, 2010, as I wrote this chapter, Paul Warren Pardus, a bus driver for disabled people, shot the orthopedic surgeon who was caring for his 84-year-old mother at Johns Hopkins Hospital. He had evidently just been told that she wasn't likely to walk again after her spinal procedure and on hearing the news, pulled a semiautomatic handgun from his waistband and shot Dr. David Cohen in the abdomen. He then ran down the hall to his mother's room and barricaded himself within with her.

Over the subsequent two hours, police secured and evacuated that por-tion of the hospital, and a SWAT team was summoned. As the predictable flurry of news reports ensued, a surge of related tweets on the topic pushed the story into the top ten list on Twitter. Eventually, after hearing nothing from the room, the police entered and found both Pardus and his mother dead with gunshot wounds to the head in a presumed murder-suicide. According to Pardus's brother, Alvin Gibson, "I guess [he did it] because he thought my mom was suffering because the surgery wasn't successful and she probably wouldn't be able to walk again. She was a dear, sweet lady. She just wanted to walk around like she did when she was younger."[1] Cohen recovered, but the news rocketed around the medical world.

Like Pardus, Latincic's husband was upset by similarly unmet expectations of the medical system, and her sons were alarmed enough to ask the police to go over and talk to their father. Hospital security also became involved. While some hospitals screen every visitor with a metal detector, most don't. Yet violence in the health-care setting is on the rise, and some experts feel that controlling access to the hospital is a critical part of the solution. Modern hospitals have increasingly become pressure cookers where doctors, nurses, patients and families grapple with tough emotional issues, critical life-and-death decisions and, sometimes, mutually incompatible goals.

By Friday afternoon of my week on service, it was clear that Mrs. Latincic was "struggling," a term I sometimes use when talking to families wanting updates about very ill loved ones in the ICU. Her medical condition had worsened to the point that we were no longer able to get a sufficient amount of oxygen into her lungs using the respirator. Her kidneys were shutting down and she was now on dialysis. She was deeply sedated and on a complicated regimen of extreme antibiotics as well as four different drugs to support her blood pressure. We measured and analyzed her urine output, liver function, cardiac performance and lungs' ability to exchange oxygen and carbon dioxide between blood and air. All of this information was stored in an intelligent intensive care electronic medical record that could display trended graphics and automatically identify aberrant laboratory values.

Dedicated doctors and nurses watched over her night and day, with assistance from a team of doctors and nurses located off-site who augmented the vigilance of the bedside team with smart software and audiovisual feeds from the room. They used a combination of computer logic and human vigilance to pick up vital sign anomalies even when the intensive care nurse wasn't in the room. Despite all of this extreme care, Mrs. Latincic deteriorated inexorably.

Eventually, there was really only one last-ditch option available to us, which was to put her on a heart-lung bypass machine that could artificially oxygenate the blood and support her heart function and blood pressure. The technical term for this intervention is *extra-corporeal membrane oxygenation,* or ECMO. It is essentially the same technology as the one we use to bypass the heart and lungs during cardiac surgical bypass grafting or transplantation. It was used to good effect in ICUs around the world during the H1N1 influenza epidemic of 2009 and 2010. Many relatively young patients actually spent weeks on ECMO while their lungs were inflamed and flooded with secretions due to the virus, and most survived.

But ECMO is an extreme intervention, very personnel-intensive and expensive. In the past, respirators fit that description, too, as did dialysis, but now we use these technologies routinely in critical care. In fact, it's not uncommon for today's intensive care teams to start dying patients on dialysis once their kidneys fail, almost as a shorthand way of demonstrating to the family that "we're doing everything medically possible"—even when the team *knows* that "doing everything" is not going to save the patient. Dialysis is not going to cure an 80-year-old woman with terminal organ failure, but we start it anyway. As a result of what might be described as short-sighted decisions like these, a significant portion of Western health-care costs are expended on hospital interventions during the terminal six months of patients' lives.

As with terminal dialysis, ECMO was equally incapable of curing Mrs. Margarita Latincic of whatever combination of autoinflammatory and infectious processes was overwhelming her kidneys, lungs, liver and heart. But I actually considered it briefly. I almost alerted the surgical team and the cardiac surgeon who would be involved in starting the heart-lung bypass should we go that route. But then I came to my senses. My patient was almost 70 years old and had an incurable illness. She had already benefited from almost 20 years of intensive medical care and three prior transplants, and we'd already thrown everything short of the kitchen sink into the mix during this present stay. I decided to not offer ECMO as an alternative.

During the span of my life, medicine's approach to end-of-life scenarios has swung from one in which the doctor often made unilateral life-and-death decisions without much input from the patient or family to today's "do everything" attitude. In my father's era, for example, it was not unheard of for a doctor to quietly prescribe a lethal dose of morphine to a patient in the very painful terminal stages of malignancy. Today we consumers have been seduced by decades of relentless medical progress and miracle stories of patients who awakened after years in a coma or survived horrific injuries after extended hospitalizations. And we providers have been trained, or sometimes sued, to undertake every conceivable and, often, previously unconceivable intervention even in the face of hopeless odds. But the balance is beginning to tip back in a more rational direction.

We are embarking on an era in which the costs and relative benefits of medical interventions will be closely scrutinized. In my hospital, we're measuring more and more how much treatment costs versus its effectiveness. We even measure patient satisfaction, how long patients stay on hold on the phone, the time to accommodate a request for an appointment, the length of time it takes for a given surgeon to do a routine operation, the number of patient complaints about each of our doctors and so on. As we computerize, it will inevitably become possible to measure more processes and outcomes. Where a doctor of my father's era felt quite comfortable starting a sentence with the words, "In my practice, I like to....," there is now a growing sense that it might be possible to identify *best* practices. In the future, we're going to see more science—and less art—in medical care.

I recently attended what's known in the software world as a Users' Group Meeting in Verona, Wisconsin, at the headquarters of a giant medical software company. Users from hospitals all over the country had come to this small town outside of Madison, the home of the giant University of Wisconsin, to see the company's latest offerings in programs designed for billing, medical records and interfaces with medical devices. While this company's campus is strikingly beautiful, with imaginative venues and fireplaces scattered throughout its building, most of its software modules have relatively dull, unimaginative names like OpTime, the software used in the operating room product; CareEverywhere, a medical record interface; or PlanLink, for providers and payer organizations.

One of the user hospitals showcased a product known as the Physician Pulse, a type of electronic dashboard showing a combination of bar graphs, trend lines and numeric cells.

As the executive physician from the hospital went through his slides, my first thought was that he was using the dashboard to illustrate the performance of his hospital, or perhaps one of the practices, relative to established quality and safety metrics, like infections. But then I got it. The Physician Pulse product was actually a dashboard designed to show the performance of a *single doctor* relative to a bunch of performance metrics—like the number of orders he wrote while the patient was still in the room, his billings and the percent he was compliant with institutionally endorsed best practices. Just like the flow sheet hanging from a sick patient's bed charting the pulse and heart beat, the flashing values on the doctor's dashboard represented the vital signs of that physician's *professional practice.* The Physician Pulse product was essentially equivalent to a medical record of the doctor.

The physician executive went on to say, with what I might only have imagined to have been a small smirk, that these indicators would *never* be used to discipline a doctor! They were merely intended to identify, in real time, doctors who were, as he put it, "struggling." Dr. Chief Medical Executive then handed the mike over to the other half of his dog-and-pony show, a stocky guy wearing a tee shirt decorated with a picture of Yoda, who prefaced his remarks with the disclaimer, "I am *not* a doctor." Mr. Tee Shirt did allow, however, that he worked with Dr. CME and that they actually met pretty regularly. Mr. TS eventually admitted to being a "data miner," and his job, he said, was to determine whether struggling doctors could be identified using performance data and then whether interventions designed by Dr. CME could be shown, with scientific rigor, to change their behavior.

Dr. CME and Mr. TS went on to spend the remainder of the hour showing examples of Physician Pulse visuals, handing mikes and laser pointers back and forth like Olympic track stars). There was nary a dropped line, or baton.

> Dr. CME: Here's a doctor who was struggling [air quotes] with getting his charts dictated on time. I intervened, and as you can see here [highlighting a bend in the curve with a red laser dot] he got better.
>
> Mr. TS: It was trivial [grins] to pull this data out of the data warehouse.
>
> Dr. CME: Here's another doctor who was struggling. You can see her decrease in productivity here [another red dot].
>
> Mr. TS: After some analysis we determined that the IT [information technology] guys had closed one of her exam rooms during this period to install a new computer. My bad [laughs].
>
> Mr. TS: One of the institutional priorities identified by leadership [air quotes] last year was to identify outlier docs with more complaints than the national norms for their discipline. We were able to mine the data to spot them.

Dr. CME: We modeled our program after the one at Vanderbilt, where they showed that high complaints correlated with a higher risk for malpractice suits. With [TS]'s help, and this data, we were able to identify those doctors who were struggling, and intervene on them [*sic*].

Whether or not one likes it, and a lot of doctors don't, this kind of data *is* being collected and analyzed, and it *will* be used to intervene. Used responsibly, moreover, it will allow hospitals to identify doctors who are not complying with appropriate requirements for timely completion of documentation, as in the first example; who are suffering from remediable practice management problems, as with the second; or who are at risk for lawsuits. And it *is* reasonable to use rigorously collected data to identify struggling doctors in much the same way that we do struggling patients. It is also appropriate for an institution to intervene in an attempt to improve the situation, exactly as we do with patients. This is all good stuff—just very foreign to traditional medical care. To be fair, similar data is being collected about practices, hospitals and health systems, as well as insurers and drug and device manufacturers; we'll soon have dashboards for all. Medical care, quality and costs will be much more transparent in the future.

Before I departed for home on Friday evening, I reviewed Mrs. Latincic's latest medical data and consulted with the night staff that would be looking after her. We talked about her status, why I had decided ECMO wasn't appropriate and what to expect in the next few hours. We had met with her sons earlier and figuratively "hung crepe," a term derived from the ancient practice of hanging black bunting over the door of the home where someone had recently died. We had, in other words, told them to expect their mother's imminent death. Yet, as often happens, we all agreed to continue to do "everything" in the meantime because, as they put it, she was a "survivor" and had pulled through a number of prior medical crises. In reality, we had exhausted our options.

Just before I left, I looked in the door of Margarita Latincic's room. A tiny, once-beautiful woman, she lay in the middle of the hospital bed with tubes running off to machines in every direction. The machines made a variety of humming, whooshing and beeping noises. Her skin had a purple-green cast. The purple resulted from poorly oxygenated blood circulating through her system; due to her malfunctioning lungs, blood that would ordinarily be rich in oxygen and therefore red, was an unhealthy purple. The greenish hue was due to too much of a yellowish liver-based pigment called bilirubin in her system. Her lungs, liver and kidneys no longer worked—these combined organ failures leave patients with skin the color of a resolving bruise. Her fingers and toes were the worst—a dark purple-black due to the medications we were using to keep her blood pressure normal; these drugs constrict the vessels in areas of vulnerable blood flow. Sometimes the fingers and toes of critical care survivors turn black and die, just as with frostbite, and eventually need amputation.

I told my fellow that I thought she would die in a matter of hours and to keep me updated. I got home, had dinner with my family and went to bed at ten. The fellow called a couple of times with questions around midnight and my "Chi Gong" ringtone woke me up for them, as designed. His calls stopped around one, however, and I slept through the rest of the night until my "Inspired Asian Morning" alarm tone rang. The text message alert hadn't awakened me at 2:50 AM, which was just as well, because the message read: "Bed nine did die. Family was at bedside and withdrew."

I presumed that meant that the sons finally recognized that death was inevitable and told the team to discontinue support—to turn off the machines. My presumption was correct. Mrs. Latincic died almost immediately. In a sense, it was a good ending. Also, my fellow had demonstrated a nice grasp of the use of modern media in medical care, calling me only for issues that required two-way communication—things I could do something about—transitioning to the one-way text message when all that was left was to inform.

The fact that I received an automatically triggered Attending Mortality Form Notification email a mere 12 minutes later, at 3:02 AM, indicated that all of the linked electronic systems were also working optimally behind the scenes. Someone at the hospital had filled out an online death certificate within moments of her death, automatically triggering an email to me, her attending physician. The Attending Mortality Form is designed to capture subjective impressions about causes of death that might not be apparent from the medical record, to help with quality improvement. There are questions like "Was this death expected?" and "Do you think the death was preventable?" There's also a free-form box that can be used to enter any "issues with the patient's care that you feel should be addressed systematically."

Our mortality report is one of many new mechanisms we've designed to gather feedback on patient care processes from the front lines. It's modeled on principles espoused by Edwards Deming, the continuous-quality-improvement guru who asked every assembly-line worker at industrial plants to suggest ways to improve workflow and products. Each death at our institution is reviewed for potential errors as well as to identify themes susceptible to improvements in process. Curiously, Deming's principles were embraced by the Japanese, who named their highest prize for business success after him, well before they came to be appreciated in his home country, the United States.

Six Sigma and lean management are two additional, now widely accepted methods for improving quality and reducing costs. Both are diffusing into medicine from Fortune 500 organizations such as Honeywell and General Electric. Six Sigma manufacturing aims to achieve greater than 99 percent defect-free production. Lean management is designed to focus a company's resources solely on the creation of value for the end customer—and in medicine, that is the patient. I even know a few doctors and nurses who are in the process of becoming Six Sigma green and black belts—experts in the application of statistical analysis and continuous quality improvement to medical processes.

In my father's era, and at the beginning of my own, if a patient like Margarita Latincic died, she just died and that was the end of it. A house officer filled out a paper death certificate, which was filed away as the last page in the medical record. Of course, in my father's era, Mrs. Latincic would have "just died" of liver failure without benefit of multiple transplants and 15 additional years of life.

The medical world is very different today. We have an unprecedented ability to measure the bodily functions of any given patient as well as all of the complicated processes of patient care. Doctors and nurses are using techniques derived from industry to measure and improve care. Of course, it's fair to inquire, "*Quis custodiet ipsos custodes?*"—a Latin phrase from the poet Juvenal that was posed to Socrates in Plato's *Republic*—which translates to "Who watches the watchmen?" Hospital administrators and safety officers are watching the clinicians. Regulatory agencies and insurers are watching the hospitals. The government is watching the insurers. And voters are watching the government.

Medical students entering the profession today will have a very different education and career than I have had. They will be taught to access information when they need to, using all of today's varied on-demand resources, rather than becoming walking medical compendiums (know-it-alls), as I was. They will be intimately familiar with the nuanced use of electronic communication devices—when to call, when to text, when to use a two-way video option like Skype or Apple's FaceTime. They will be confronted with patient care and ethical issues as I was when I briefly considered ECMO— situations where "more" is not the same as "better." They'll grapple with the inappropriately inflated expectations of family members like Mr. Latincic and Paul Warren Pardus, the man who shot his doctor before killing his sick mother and then himself. They'll care for a patient population in which a much of the disease burden is due to discretionary, unhealthy lifestyle choices like smoking, poor diet, insufficient exercise, too much alcohol, unprotected sex and drug use.

Today's medical students will also have to choose between sexy careers in sub-sub-specialties, like transplant surgery or transplant infectious disease, versus less glamorous primary care careers that the government would like to see more of to resolve the current serious shortage. They'll be much more familiar with the use of numbers and statistics in the administration of care; and they'll aspire to *best* practices, rather than attempting to find some personalized alternative peculiar to their own reading of the literature. This new generation of physicians will not bridle at being measured and compared with other practitioners, because that's the future of medicine. There won't be an alternative.

CHAPTER 2

BONES

In one of the best episodes of the iconic, long-running science fiction series *Star Trek,* the ship's physician, Dr. Leonard McCoy, nicknamed "Bones," is called upon to examine a sick man on the outpost. He concludes, "Heartbeat is all wrong...temperature is...[he pauses], Jim, this man is a *Klingon.*" Dr. McCoy reaches this conclusion after examining the patient with his portable, universal diagnostic device, the tricorder.

While the tricorder was a figment of Gene Roddenberry's (the series creator) imagination in the 1960s, and today's doctors still carry stethoscopes, ophthalmoscopes and goniometers, we are getting closer to having an all-in-one portable diagnostic tool. This gadget is today's smartphone. Many of the features that *Star Trek*'s writers attributed to Dr. McCoy's utility tool are now emerging from mobile device app stores. Apps, of course, are the ubiquitous cellphone programs like the ones used on Apple's iPhone.

Like many urban hospitals, particularly the older ones, my hospital is a sprawling hodgepodge of buildings that seem to have been thrown together almost randomly. The external architecture varies from one to the next, the first floor of one is sometimes level with the second of another and the connections between any two are not always obvious. We've spent a lot of time and thought on helping patients and families find their way around; yet every time I walk the corridors, I find some poor person or couple lost at an intersection, peering at the maps. They're invariably trying to figure out which way to go for a radiology or lab study, or where to find a sick loved one.

A lot of people move through the hospital's halls and across its bridges every day. A lot of business gets done in these hallways and overpasses as well. Trainees brief faculty members about the next patient they'll see while the team moves through corridors from one floor to the next, and the consulting faculty members, in return, dispense clinical pearls of wisdom. In fact, as the pace of medicine has increased in modern times, many doctors, to be efficient, spend much of their time in some form of communication while they move from one location to the next.

In my father's era, doctors could only be reached by overhead loudspeaker "paging" messages. A suite of operators fielded calls originating in and outside the hospital. They consulted loose-leaf binders to determine who was on call for a given service and paged that person. Each page operator—and they were inevitably female in that era—had her own distinctive voice: her handle. Some voices were huskier than others, and many had distinctive regional accents or styles: "Dr. Han-ssson...Dr. Will-ih-am Han-ssson...plee-zuh di-yul the ahhp-er-ay-tor." And on the rare occasion that I met one of these ladies, they never looked the way I had imagined— invariably quite different from what their voices had suggested.

Back then, one could see doctors up and down the hospital's long corridors, even a long way off in the distance, cock an ear to better hear whenever the overhead operator spoke. Telephones were scattered at frequent intervals along the halls to shorten the distance and time it took to respond. Extra-long cords were often stretched to the limit between the handset and the base unit in the cafeteria, as maxed-out house staff tried to simultaneously pay for food and answer a nurse's question on a phone located some distance from the cashier.

In the late 1970s, electronic pagers first became available, and the earliest adopters were physicians. By wearing a beeper in that era, you were clearly labeling yourself as a doctor. Single friends of mine wore their pagers out in public as ostentatiously as possible. Paging technology matured, and by the early 1990s, wide-area messaging became possible. At that point the value of these devices immediately expanded to other industries in which workers were geographically dispersed, and a given individual carrying a beeper on a belt might equally well be a doctor, a plumber or a drug dealer. The appeal of a beeper plummeted.

Passive, receive-only technology was eventually supplanted by two-way pagers, so that a "pagee" could communicate a text message back to the originating pager. The pager's range increased from regional to national, and transmitter-receiver units shrank. Then, the first brick-sized portable cell phones became available in the 1990s, albeit with limited battery life, range and fidelity.

Today, pagers are almost obsolete. Most hospitals issue loaner cell phones equipped with messaging software to incoming residents. More-senior staff carry some brand of smartphone. In fact, market researchers believe we're at the cusp of a revolutionary change in the way physicians go about looking for information. Monique Levy, an expert health-care industry analyst, predicts that by 2012, "All physicians will walk around with a stethoscope and a smart mobile device, and there will be very few professional activities that physicians won't be doing on their handhelds. Physicians will be going online first for the majority of their professional needs and will be regularly pulling online resources into patient consultations."[1]

In hospital hallways every day, physicians pass by, oblivious to their surroundings, heads down, smartphones held like a precious fragile creature in their upturned palms even though they're merely reading email, texting messages or looking up references. While the older doctors struggle with the size of the text and peer at the screen through the bottom portion of their bifocals, younger trainees thumb-type messages, rapid-fire, like secretaries of yore.

High-technology medical care depends on tight, real-time communication about rapidly evolving situations. My fellow was able to stay in close touch with me about the course of Mrs. Latincic's worsening situation as I walked from the hospital to the car, drove to my home and lay in bed that night. The advent of cell phones and smartphones has changed the nature of medical care in substantial ways. Whereas providers at the bedside—the nurses and trainees—might once have had to wait for direction while an expert could be located (perhaps on a golf course), she's now immediately reachable by portable phone. Of course, once the connection is made, the nurse or resident still needs to describe the situation to the expert, and the expert has to rely on the provider for information. And unreliable information can lead to trouble.

I have been misled by well-intentioned but inexperienced bedside providers whose description of a patient sounded dramatically more dire, or, even worse, rosier, than the one I found when I eventually arrived. But that, too, is about to change. The expert will soon be able to see exactly what's happening at the bedside with information fed directly to his phone or tablet computer from bedside monitors, laboratory computers, radiology imaging software and cameras that allow direct videoconferencing with nurses, residents, colleagues, families or patients themselves.

The adoption of cell phones has accelerated the pace of medicine. Also, the different spheres of medicine are more interlocked. Whereas a primary physician used to write a referral for an appointment with a specialist, expecting it not to happen until two weeks later, now primary care physicians want to get information or take action quickly. They have a question about someone who's in the office, and they need an answer immediately. An emergency room physician may need to find a doctor to help with a critically ill patient while there's still time to intervene and preserve brain function, heart muscle or a life. If he knows he can call for assistance day or night, and that someone will immediately pick up the phone every time, he'll send more patients into the care of that very responsive doctor. Granting access to oneself is an evolutionary adaptation for a physician—the equivalent of the opposable thumb—in a professional environment that's rapidly becoming faster-paced and more competitive.

Cell phones are also a conduit to important information. Dog-eared copies of what we called the *PDR*, shorthand for the *Physicians' Desk Reference*, were available at every nursing station in every hospital a decade ago. The book is still updated annually, and over 60 editions have been printed to date. It is a comprehensive encyclopedia of drug information, showing generic and brand names, pictures, dosages and side effects for nearly every available drug approved by the Food and Drug Administration (FDA). But the book is more than 3,000 pages long and weighs about seven pounds. Today, questions about a drug can be answered much more readily with a quick search on a smartphone. Mobile devices can access an entire medical library of information in seconds. As Levy, the medical analyst, suggests, we've reached a tipping point where physicians are equally likely to use their phone or a hard-copy reference work to find needed information about a medical topic.

Levy's 2012 prediction has it only half right: tomorrow's physicians will certainly "walk around with a...smart mobile device," but they may not even carry a stethoscope. Their smart mobile device may be loaded with apps that substitute for many of today's signature medical diagnostic tools.

The smartphone itself can already be used as a stethoscope. Its microphone can be placed against the chest or abdominal wall to pick up sounds emanating from deep within the body. One application has programmed "wizards" that can be used by the novice to diagnose different sounds based on the location, audio characteristics and type of sound. The program uses sound filtering and noise canceling features that amplify distant heart sounds. Previously these special sound-processing features were available only on expensive, high-end stethoscopes, but now they're built in to this inexpensive smartphone application.

I recently downloaded iStethoscope Expert (a product of Current Clinical Strategies), one of several stethoscope apps from the medical section of the Apple store. It's advertised as a way to employ one's iPhone as an electronic stethoscope. In fact, there are many uses for the application—it comes equipped with an acoustic library of normal and abnormal heart, lung and bowel sounds. When the user selects a given example, like the cardiac "quadruple gallop," the phone cues up a movie (using QuickTime, Apple's proprietary media player) that shows an acoustic trace of the sound and plays the accompanying audio. The term quadruple gallop describes a cardiac rhythm in which there are four, rather than the usual two, *lub-dub* sounds with each heartbeat. It is reminiscent of the hoofbeats of a horse at full tilt and suggests that the patient has severe heart failure. Whereas medical students, nurses or paramedical trainees might have the opportunity to hear this sound in a real patient only once or twice during the course of their education, they can listen to the app's example over and over until they've got it down pat.

The iStethoscope Expert library contains a suite of more than 60 different murmurs, rubs, gallops, clicks and rumbles characteristic of different heart problems. A collection of lung and bowel sounds also provides brief descriptions, phonocardiograms and audiograms of each. There are old favorites like pulmonary "whispered pectoriloquy" and "egophony," and bowel "borborygmi," "tinkles" and "rushes." There's even a spooky recording of the "death rattle" described so often in old books—the ones that were written back in the day when ordinary people died ordinary deaths—at home. (The mind reels thinking of how they went about recording the rattle.) Used purely for its acoustic medical library function, this app has merit; but there's much, much more!

An additional, extremely novel feature is the ability to record a patient's heartbeat or lung sounds "for the record," for comparison over time—even for analysis by someone else or by some next-generation computer with heartbeat recognition software. This opens up a world of interesting and previously unimaginable possibilities. A patient's heart, lung and bowel sounds could, for example, easily be recorded into a medical record with each physical examination. For example, a primary care physician might record a worrisome exam and send it in an email to a consulting cardiologist.

The app's designers may have anticipated that this kind of software might not win immediate acceptance within the brotherhood of medicine. So they hedged their bets by putting in a few additional features to win over nonmedical app shoppers who weren't sufficiently enticed by the ability to play doctor with their iPhone on themselves or, perhaps more enticingly, on others. This iPhone app can actually "listen through walls!" What teenage boy could pass *this* up?

Perhaps the canniest sales pitch on the iStethoscope Expert developer's descriptive website promotes an approach expert obstetricians have used to reassure their patients since the invention of the stethoscope by Laennec back in the early 1800s. With this $1.99 smartphone application, an anxious mother or father, or any soon-to-be parent for that matter, can have peace of mind. They can listen to baby's heartbeat—anytime they feel the need!

I tried this application on myself. When I used the phone's speaker to project the sound, all I got was a screeching wail of feedback. But when I used earbuds, as the company recommends, I could actually hear lung sounds quite well, as well as the rumblings of my stomach as it churned away on my lunch. It was harder to hear heart sounds, but the company also sells a stethoscope attachment that can be plugged into the bottom of the iPhone and that's better suited to cardiac examination.

In its current form, the stethoscope app is not yet suitable for true medical use, but it isn't at all hard to imagine a version that would work just as well as or better than today's traditional medical instruments. Considering the capabilities of sophisticated music-recognition apps like Shazam and Soundhound that can identify the singer, title and composer of most music after a sample of only a few bars, one can readily envision something comparable for medical care.

The iStethoscope Expert isn't the only smartphone app designed to duplicate or demystify the magical things that only doctors were privy to until recently. MIT researchers have designed NETRA, the Near Eye Tool for Refractive Assessment, to reproduce the techniques ophthalmologists and optometrists use to determine the prescription that a patient needs. With a specially designed mobile phone add-on piece, a nonspecialist can determine how much refraction is needed to correct the vision of a near- or farsighted individual.

The patient looks through a lens at the phone's screen and uses the phone's controls to move parallel red and green lines closer and closer until they overlap. Depending on the degree of curvature of the eye lens, the overlap point will vary among individuals. The same process is repeated eight times, as the lines are rotated sequentially through 360 degrees to form a complete representation of the patient's lens. Once the measurements are complete, special software calculates the prescription necessary to correct vision in that eye. The same process is performed for the other eye, and, with that data, a pair of corrective lenses can be made.

A UCLA professor, Aydogan Ozcan, and his group have developed a lens-free microscope weighing less than two ounces and designed to attach to most camera-based cell phones.[2] Unlike traditional lens-based microscopes, the images in these inexpensive devices (less than $10) are captured using a process known as diffraction, which permits the reconstruction of an image from the shadows that it casts. A light-emitting diode shines through a blood or saliva specimen, and because the cellular elements in the sample are semi-transparent, both the cells and their subcellular elements cast shadows. The shadows are reconstructed into holographic images of the cells, which can then be transmitted from the field to a pathologist in some remote location, usually a hospital laboratory, for analysis.

This technology will soon be deployed in Africa, where cell phones are plentiful but pathologists are sparse. Ozcan's work has been supported by the Gates Foundation, National Geographic and the National Science Foundation. Samples, such as blood smears, can quickly be loaded onto single-use chips that slide into the microscope; and because of the large aperture of the sensor array, no special alignment or cleaning techniques are necessary—which makes this technology ideal for field use by relatively untrained workers. Malaria is an example of a disease widely prevalent in Africa for which this technique is particularly suitable. A drop of blood can be applied to this "lab on a chip," and the malarial parasites are easily identifiable.

While telemedical analysis usually is done by an expert who analyzes an image sent using text messaging or email, Ozcan's group has also developed an algorithm for local use. This is essentially an app that identifies and counts red cells, white cells and microparticles like bacteria or parasites, permitting instantaneous on-site reports.

It is easy to imagine that cell-based technologies being developed for impoverished areas might eventually come to be used in medically well-served countries. The technology will improve, the cost will decrease, and the old methods will eventually be displaced by cheaper new ones.

In another novel application of smartphones to medicine that was described in the *Washington Post,* Vishal Giare did what many other neighbors of other medical workers do: he consulted his friend Dr. Neal Sikka after Giare's four-year-old son, Rohan, cut the bridge of his nose.[3] At the time, little Rohan was doing something that I've been unable to keep my own sons from doing—jumping on the bed. But rather than walking the bloodied boy to his neighbor's house, Giare snapped a picture of the cut with his Blackberry and sent it to Sikka, an emergency physician. He took a look at the photo and recommended a trip to the ER for stitches rather than a Band-Aid. Dr. Sikka is now studying whether he can accurately predict whether or not a cut needs suturing based on cell-phone photos plus a questionnaire (about the most recent tetanus vaccine, for example) that could be answered on the same device. While it would be useful to know when it is appropriate to go to an emergency room for help, many of my friends would be just as happy to know when they *don't* have to go and sit for hours in an overcrowded ER, only to find that a bandage is all that's needed.

The resolution, autofocus and autoflash capabilities of cell phone cameras have dramatically improved, making the images much more useful for interpretation by remote experts, who can use image-enhancement techniques on their own computers to acquire additional information. Two-way videochat technologies like Apple's FaceTime will soon open up a whole *new* avenue of possibilities for consultations between one provider and another or between provider and patient.

Fujitsu has developed communication standards for medical devices and cell phones.[4] The Fujitsu phone uses the Bluetooth wireless protocol to gather information from similarly equipped machines that measure blood pressure, heart rate, blood sugar and weight. While these phones are intended to store and forward the data to doctors at remote locations, the next wave of apps will allow a patient to record, interpret and analyze his *own* data. We're likely to see much more in the way of applications that allow each of us as patients to have greater control over the acquisition of useful data for preventative and chronic health care.

As of this writing, there are already more than 6,000 medical or health applications in Apple's App Store, and the numbers increase every day. Many of these apps are focused on the consumer rather than the provider. There are apps to track caloric intake, exercise and weight. These might reduce the necessity for weight-loss programs or change how we approach health education. There are specific applications allowing diabetics to follow their blood levels of a diabetic marker called *hemoglobin A1c*. These apps can track the individual patient over time, as well as the individual patient compared to others with the same disease in the same geographic area.

I've worked on another cell phone application with Lingraphica, a company developing tools to help patients with various forms of aphasia, the medical term for speech difficulties resulting from brain injuries. Aphasia is profoundly frustrating for patients who may experience it after a stroke or injury to the speech areas of the brain. They know what they want to say but can't say it. Lingraphica has an app that allows patients to quickly find a picture of the object they want, but for which they can't locate the word. The patient can then use the picture or a linked audio description to communicate his needs to someone else.

In the past, I thought of aphasia as an inconvenient problem for patients who had recovered from a devastating stroke. But I now have several friends or relatives who've experienced injuries that affected their speech in some way. My friend Ron had a profound but ultimately reversible injury to what's known as Broca's area in the brain. Patients with damage to this very specific anatomical area on the left side of the brain know exactly what they want to say, but can't get it out.

Ron had developed an aneurysm and bleeding in the brain. The aneurysm was corrected, and CT and MRI scans showed no permanent damage. Still, he continued to have problems with coordination and speech. One major, persistent problem was his inability to express what he wanted to say. He'd start with, "I need to ... I need to ..." and then stop, completely unable to find the word he wanted. He'd try again and again without success. The frustration and anger were obvious—to the point that he'd hit the bed rails with his hands. Eventually he'd stop trying and turn away.

He eventually recovered enough to go to a rehabilitative facility and then home. He's now totally recovered from this life-threatening event, and we've had a chance to talk about the whole illness with the benefit of some distance from it. Ron's a bright, articulate and thoughtful man, and he loves to talk. He'd gone through a lot during his hospitalization, but he said that the aphasia, and the frustration of being unable to communicate was the worst thing he'd ever experienced in his entire life.

The Lingraphica cell phone app, had we been able to use it, would have made communication much easier. What's more, there's good evidence to show that continuous use of the smartphone app serves as an electronic speech pathologist, helping to rewire the brain's connections. My work with the company has involved the extension of this tool for use in patients on ventilators in the intensive care unit. While most of these individuals don't have brain injuries, they're equally unable to communicate their needs because of the breathing tube in their mouths.

Asthmapolis is another application integrating a cell phone and a smart asthma inhaler. It tracks when and where a patient used medication or experienced symptoms. The application can remind a patient that a scheduled med is due, it can be used as a diary of symptoms and it can keep a GPS-based map of problem locations. From personal experience, I know that my allergy symptoms are worse in certain parts of the country during certain seasons.

Cell phone medical tools are new, and the ways in which they'll be used in medicine are evolving all the time. To be sure, innovative physicians are already using smartphones for expert advice and for applications that facilitate charting and prescribing. But it's clear that some of the most innovative mobile tools will come from consumer-oriented products, or from tools originally designed as inexpensive alternatives to traditional devices.

Medical students now live at the cutting edge of technology. They are extremely savvy about new paradigms, transitioning smoothly from telephone to text to social networks, while their medical teachers are often much less comfortable with the era of electronic communications. Today's students will begin their careers just as electronic health records become prevalent. And they'll help to define the best ways to use these new tools that will dramatically alter the delivery and consumption of health care, right before our eyes.

CHAPTER 3

SEE YA, IN 2015

On a recent crisp autumn day I watched a new crop of students matricu-lating into the oldest medical school in the country—the University of Pennsylvania's ("Penn's") School of Medicine. It was founded nearly two-and-a-half centuries ago, in 1765, a decade before America claimed its inde-pendence; and, as we'll see later in the book, the school's founders were intimately involved in the American Revolution.

While it seemed like it should have been an ancient rite, as we'll see this white-coat ceremony is actually a young tradition. By donning the short white coat at the ceremony, just as I had done years earlier, the class of 2014 was symbolically and officially being inducted as the most junior members of the ancient profession of medicine.

As I watched, I wondered who were these young people who had chosen to go into a medical career at a time when many of my mid-career colleagues are feeling constrained, harried and pessimistic about their own future. Were these new students working with some outdated view of the world? Were they like those last few wannabe gunslingers who must have boarded a train headed West at the end of the nineteenth century toward a frontier that was already over? Or will they be the ones who bring a new medical future, one in which the aging old coots of my generation sit rocking in our meta-phorical medical rocking chairs, scratching our scrawny, unshaven chins and crowing, "That'll never work…"?

These newest members of the medical profession were, I learned, a multiracial, multinational group of men and women, mostly in their mid-twenties. Some wore suits while others were casual, wearing sports jackets, with or without ties, and khakis, or, in the case of some of the women, short, startlingly revealing summer dresses. By the end of the ceremony, 163 students from 24 states would make the transition, filling an entire section of the auditorium with a monochromatic snowy sea of white.

Upon stepping onto the stage, each student was handed a coat emblazoned with the university's logo, and, having donned the coat, each walked to the center of the stage and stepped up to a podium to address the packed house of family and friends. They introduced themselves, said something about their educational background and invariably spoke some words of thanks. Most acknowledged parents and siblings; many mentioned boyfriends, girlfriends or spouses; one even spoke directly to the admissions staff, thanking them for their endorsement.

Their voices ranged from soprano to bass and from mousy to booming. Some obviously relished the spotlight. One tall, bushy-headed young man, whose white coat didn't quite reach his wrists, bounded up to the stand and nearly shouted, "I *am* the most interesting man in the world," paraphrasing a bearded adventurer in a popular beer commercial. Others in the group were clearly less enthusiastic about public speaking and mumbled into the microphone.

It was an extraordinarily disciplined group of young adults who'd arrived at Penn's medical school at the end of the summer of 2010. Most had gotten A's in the majority of their classes since the very beginning of high school. Many had passed up the "easier path" because they were preparing even then for admission to medical school years later, an outcome that wasn't by any means guaranteed, despite their hard work. Some, however, had started off in an entirely different direction and only changed course when they were well downstream. These aspirants were forced to swim very hard against the current to get to their newly chosen destination.

John Pryor's life had been like this. John's medical education started several decades prior to the white-coat ceremony that I recently attended. On June 16, 1999, when he was already a doctor, John made a videotape describing the pivotal period of his life years before. In the video he is sitting in an empty apartment, about to move to a new city, and he is the father of a young girl. He'd propped up one of those clunky old digital tape cameras on a table and pointed at himself as he sat on the last few boxes of books and bric-a-brac. In the tape, he is unshaven, looks tired, and is wearing the kind of clothing you wouldn't mind getting dirty in. The walls behind him are bare and scuffed. But he's happy. When he recorded this video memoir, John was on the way to join his family in Philadelphia.

As he puts it: "Now, with Danielle [his new baby girl], things are so much more fun. It makes you think about what the future holds for her. When she is 33, since I'm 33 now, I'll be lucky to be alive, at 66. But she'll have a very different world to live in."[1]

John had done well in high school, with a 93-percent average. After being wait-listed at Binghamton, one of New York's state universities, he was eventually admitted. He obviously enjoyed college. He called his mother at one point early on and said, "Thank you! Thank you for sending me here! This is like a country club!"

But he later admits in the video, "I didn't put the effort into college that I should have, and that's the regret part, the part that, to this day, I am regretful that I didn't put 100-percent effort into that academic side of college."

He continues, "I did, however, learn a lot. What separated me from most of the other students was that I was genuinely interested in the material. I would read textbooks and I would read the material, but I never...I have a hard time getting up in the morning, that's one thing...I never went to class before twelve. I wasn't interested in doing quizzes and labs and things I didn't think were pertinent to the material."

It's interesting now to hear him say that he had a hard time getting up in the morning, given the career path he eventually followed. Of course, John had an extracurricular, nonintramural activity that may have served as an additional distraction: he was an apprentice paramedic and traveled with the ambulance crews when he could take shifts.

He did read, however—voraciously, as it turned out. He was also a good writer and eventually wrote very compellingly about his experiences. John was self-taught and, as he put it, "read a lot of the textbooks on my own because I didn't go to class. So I did wind up learning a lot about, about everything, biochemistry, history, philosophy. But it didn't translate into good grades."

When graduation loomed, John was at a bit of a loss: "I had mixed feelings about what to do with my life. I knew that because of the paramedic work I really liked working with patients. I really liked being a paramedic and doing things. But I also enjoyed biochemistry, and I recall thinking, foolishly, that I would want to be a chemist or organic chemist or biochemist when those things were not interesting to me."

At that point on the tape, John stops for a moment, leaves the frame and then comes back to say, "I also have gotten much fatter than I was in college."

I forgot to mention that. He does look a little chubby as he sat on those boxes reminiscing about the choices he did and didn't make. He had started a branch of College Republicans, through which he met Senators Dick Lugar and Bob Dole, as well as Pat Robertson and George Bush Sr. By the end of his college years, he knew he was "a good bullshitter" with a low grade-point average and no clear way forward. His had not, to date, been a purpose-driven life. He did, it turned out, have some vague idea even then about going to medical school, but he lost track of the dates and missed the application deadlines.

I don't think of John as an egotistical guy, but he does allow that he went to one job interview, and "I just told them how great I was, and I was as good as any paramedic. Man, I remember their faces looking at me like, 'Who the fuck is this guy?' I really blew that interview and, of course, didn't get the job."

Eventually he landed in New York at Columbia University, which has a post-baccalaureate, premed program for people like John who are interested in medicine but hadn't made the right decisions at the right time. Columbia University is one of many schools that offer this kind of curriculum, which can last as short as 18 months or as long, in some cases, as five years for students who go through the program part-time. Like many, Columbia's pre-med, post-bac is very competitive, and most applicants have both high SAT scores and GPAs.

Columbia's post-bac grads are a formidable group; the school's home page features several of them. There's a Princeton graduate, a creative writing major who had worked as a veterinary assistant but hadn't realized she wanted to go to medical school until after graduation. It wasn't the veterinary experience that changed her life; she had a brother with kidney disease and eventually decided to donate one of her own kidneys to her sibling so that he could live a life without dialysis. After going through the donation process and interacting with the doctors and nurses of the transplant team, she decided she wanted to become a doctor herself. Another had been a working science writer with a graduate degree in journalism, but after an accident that necessitated surgery, she decided to practice science rather than write about it. A third was a classical violinist who'd decided to try to integrate music and healing in a medical career; he'd won a MacArthur Foundation "Genius Grant."

The Columbia curriculum basically consists of intensive remedial sciences. In the fall of the two-year continuum there are general chemistry, calculus and physics. The spring semester consists of more chemistry and more physics, and there's a summer course on statistics. Parenthetically, it's very possible to get through an entire career in medicine without understanding the first thing about chemistry, physics, calculus or statistics (don't ask me how I know). One could make a compelling argument that courses in economics, politics and psychology are better preparation. But the "hard" sciences are the traditional prerequisites for application to medical school.

Columbia's second-year curriculum moves on to the more medically relevant topics of biology and organic chemistry, with labs in both. It isn't until the summer after the second year that students take the dreaded Medical College Admission Test, commonly called the MCATs. If one takes this traditional two-year curriculum, it is actually three years before one has finished all of the requirements, including the MCATs, to apply to medical school.

There's also a five-year part-time alternative. But John Pryor didn't go to *any* of Columbia's post-bac programs. The fine print in the frequently asked questions portion of their website states: "The curriculum is designed to meet the needs of college graduates who have decided to pursue a medical education, but have taken none or only some of the basic science courses required for admission to medical school. *It is not designed to help improve the records of people who have already completed the requirements.*"

No, John ended up working as a tech in a lab at Columbia. At first he liked it. But then, "in about six months into that job, I was definitely sure I didn't want to [do] research my whole life. The lab was killing me. It was just doldrums every day. I remember I couldn't wait to get out of that place. I would cross off the days; I would cross off half the day right before I went off to lunch, and I would cross off the other half just like I was some convict in prison. And I really couldn't wait to leave that job."

He eventually moved from New York City to Albany, took a job running an electrocardiography lab and started a program teaching high school graduates how to become EKG technicians. It "was about as close to running a day care center as I ever did." But he enjoyed it, despite frustrations that got to be so awful that he shattered a beeper against a wall after covering one too many nights for people who didn't show up at work. About the same time, he also went back to working as a paramedic. At some point during that period, the light went on; he decided to go to medical school, for real this time. While his grades were "horrendous," he finally knew what he wanted—no, *needed*—to do.

"In my mind I knew that if I was given a chance,...I could do it. It was that I hadn't given any effort in anything before. And all I needed was somebody to give me that avenue to give me a try.

"I remember going to the interview at (a little hospital) in New York, some rinky-dink hospital, and we talked a little while and finally I said, I told the lady, 'You know, I'm at the absolute end of my rope. I['ve] got to get in to this school.' I would see my future, like, to July of that year. And then I would look and it would all be white, empty. I saw no future in my life until the end of medical school. It wasn't like I was depressed or anything. It was that there was no other option. I had spent a lot of time in my life trying to figure out what to do, and when I came up with the idea of medicine, when I settled on the idea that I needed to be a physician, there was no other option."

I mention John as I write about the white coat ceremony because he entered medical school during the era that these ceremonies proliferated. Most schools formalized the ceremony in the 1990s. These rituals did not proceed from some thoughtful discussion about a warm new way to welcome new practitioners into the profession—medical students have historically been the lowliest of apprentices. The first white-coat ritual occurred at the University of Chicago in 1989, prompted by the complaint of a professor who found medical students "showing up in shorts and baseball caps" for sessions "where the patients are pouring their hearts out."[2]

The school's then dean of admissions, Dr. Norma Wagoner, chose a novel solution. She designed a remedial ceremony where students were given white coats. She told her charges that "for any session where we have patients present, we expect you to look like professionals, wear the white coat and behave appropriately."[3] In other words, "Act like a grown-up."

Columbia University's College of Physicians and Surgeons formalized their white-coat ceremony in 1993 as a part of the medical school matriculation process. The ceremony was designed by and supported with funds from the Arnold P. Gold Foundation for "fostering humanism in medicine."[4] At that time, Gold was a prominent pediatric neurologist at Columbia who had noted, with dismay, a trend in the school's trainees toward scientific and technological interventions and advances, which he believed was at the expense of attention to the ill, suffering or dying patient.

Working with his wife, Sandra, colleagues at Columbia, medical educators and community leaders, Gold formed his foundation in 1988, to nurture and preserve the tradition of the caring physician. The organization set about its work by asking several questions. The first was: "Is it possible to identify candidates for medical schools who are both scientifically proficient *and* compassionate?" They also asked: "Are we already selecting idealistic and humanistic young people for medical schools and then, through the medical education process, discouraging their spirit of caring?" And: "If young doctors are *not* naturally sensitive, can we train them to be so?"[5]

With these fundamental questions in mind, the Gold Foundation distilled them into more actionable issues, such as: "What can we actually *do* to address the need for greater compassion in medical care?" "Who are the populations we want to influence?" And "How could we promote humanistic values within those populations?" The foundation targeted three distinct medical populations: students in the four years of medical school, residents and medical faculty. They concentrated their interventions on efforts fostering values that reflect humanism—empathy, respect, caring, integrity and service—and on changing behaviors so that humanism was a principal focus of medical education.

Here again, one might assume that these values have always been taught as part of the medical curriculum, but humanism per se wasn't taught explicitly until relatively recently. True, specific faculty definitely acted as role models, and some took particular pains to make sure we understood how to act as professionals, but nobody used the term "humanism" during my training. Nonetheless, a few examples stand out for me even today, decades later, as crystal-clear, succinct lessons in how to be professional and take care of patients.

Martie McCartney was the head nurse on one of the floors of the hospital, and she ran it with an iron fist in a velveteen glove. I, on the other hand, was a long-haired medical student who had grown up around hospitals in the unkempt 1970s. Unlike most of the other students, for me medical wards had been a kind of second home as I accompanied my father on weekend rounds while growing up.

One day during medical school, I walked up directly from classes to the ward that Martie ran to review information on a patient's chart. I was still wearing jeans, my customary classroom uniform. Martie knew my father, who was at that time a senior member of the medical school faculty, and she recognized me. Despite that, she dismissed me from the floor that day and told me to come back when I was dressed appropriately.

Like the professor at the University of Chicago who was put off by shorts and baseball caps, Martie believed that professionals, even professionals-in-training, should be held to a high standard of dress and comportment. She also knew that my father, who was invariably clad formally when in the hospital, would back her if I complained. Martie and I have laughed about this ever since, but the lesson stuck.

A second lesson came from Dr. Truman Schnabel, who was known to his friends as "Nipper." Dr. Schnabel took several of us into a patient's room on rounds one day, where he talked to the woman and carefully examined her. In the process he had to move her food tray out of the way, pull down the bedcovers and undo her hospital gown. His examination was thorough but respectfully attentive to any feelings of modesty she might have felt in a room full of strangers. Dr. Schnabel passed his stethoscope under the gown when possible, or exposed only her belly while covering everything else to feel the liver and spleen.

When it came time to leave, unlike many of my other professors, Schnabel carefully retied her gown and drew the bedcovers up in the way he had found them. He then wheeled the table with her food and phone back next to the bed. He said a few reassuring words to summarize, and we left. Once in the hallway, Dr. Schnabel reviewed what he'd found on exam and headed off for the next patient, but then he stopped with an afterthought. He turned to us and said: "You should always leave the patient just the way you found her," because, he said, "it is respectful." This was how rounds went with that wonderful man.

Another famous doctor had a different approach to making his patients feel that they were the most important encounter of his day. Isidor S. Ravdin was a world-renowned University of Pennsylvania general surgeon who commanded the 20th General Hospital, one of Penn's base hospitals stationed in India during World War II. Ravdin was a master physician, a brilliant administrator and a very busy man. He was a friend of President Dwight Eisenhower and actually treated him for ileitis—inflammation of a portion of the small bowel. After the war, Ravdin returned to Philadelphia, and the university, as a Major General in the Army, in 1956. He finished his career at

Penn. Fittingly, one of the University's still-standing hospital buildings, one of that hodgepodge of structures, is named after him.

Ravdin was short and stout and sported a precise, pencil-thin moustache that must have taken extra time when shaving. He wore a blue blazer over surgical scrub clothing as he walked to and from the operating room, a habit some imitators at Penn continue to this day. It's an odd look, and strangely formal. And Ravdin smoked—a lot. Many physicians from that era smoked, including my father. In fact, cigarette companies actually advertised their wares for a time with slogans like "More Doctors Smoke Camels than any other Cigarette."[6] When I was in medical school, the surgeons' lounge outside the locker room was still a hazy room full of ashtrays where doctors would catch a smoke and a chat between cases. Several of the most prominent doctors of the era later died of smoking-related cancers of the lungs or vocal cords.

Dr. Ravdin actually died of vascular disease, almost certainly as a result of his smoking habit; but he had figured out a way to use the cigarette as a very positive, albeit subliminal, message to his charges. He'd enter a patient's room while on rounds, pull out a pack while he was talking, carefully select a cigarette, light it and sit on the side of the sickbed to chat. He didn't actually stay very long, but he crushed out each butt before leaving the room, thereby giving the impression that he'd stayed for the full smoke. The studied act of lighting up explicitly conveyed the message that he had all the time in the world for that single patient. In a letter written during the war, Ravdin said of his own life, "Each day is full but a rewarding one."[7]

Some have criticized white-coat ceremonies as being self-promotional or self-congratulatory rituals designed to emphasize the power and elitism associated with wearing a professional uniform. The Gold Foundation, on the other hand, suggests that this act of recognition and the rituals are powerful ways to imbue new students with a sense of mission and responsibility. This latter view has clearly carried the day, as white-coat ceremonies are now performed in almost every osteopathic and traditional medical school in the country at some point during the educational continuum. In fact, the idea has caught on at dental, podiatric, pharmacy, physical therapy, physician assistant and advanced nursing programs and at chiropractic schools as well.

Fifty-one percent of the students entering Penn's class of 2014 were women, and they ranged in age from a very precocious 20 to the mid-thirties. A quarter of the class were underrepresented minorities, and almost

20 percent were Asian. Students hailed from over 60 different colleges scattered across the United States; and while most had majored in one of the sciences, fully one-third had majored in some nonscientific field. A significant majority had taken a year or more off between college and medical school. These non-premed and delayed-entry scholars, like John Pryor, bring interesting backgrounds and viewpoints to what might otherwise be a more narrowly focused student body—Penn looks very favorably on applicants with this background.

Many had also spent time working in community service of some kind. Some had tutored inner-city children. Others worked in soup kitchens, Habitat for Humanity or homeless shelters. They had worked with troubled adolescents, teen mothers, the Red Cross, Big Brother programs and domestic and international clinics or hospitals in Africa, South America, China, Australia or Europe. There were athletes and musicians, scientists, high-school teachers and political campaign staffers from both the Obama and Clinton 2008 campaigns.

Seventeen percent of the incoming students were headed toward medical research, pursuing a six-year combined MD-PhD track. While it takes longer than the traditional four-year curriculum, this track puts its graduates at a significant advantage when it comes time to prepare for NIH-funded research. The students included a Fulbright scholar, National Science Foundation grantees, and fellows of the National Institutes of Health and the Howard Hughes Medical Institute.

It was clear by the time the last student stepped up to speak at the 2010 white-coat ceremony that this was an extraordinary group of young people. Dr. Gail Morrison, the senior vice dean for education, concluded her introductory remarks by saying, "We look for students who bring a well-rounded perspective and a range of experience as well as scientific understanding to the study of medicine. I look forward to seeing the incoming class of 2010 progress, and to the unique contributions they will make to medicine."[8]

When John Pryor was finally ready to apply for medical school, although he was definitely well rounded and had "perspective and a range of experience," his application wouldn't have made the first cut of Penn's admissions committee. It wouldn't have made any sense for him to spend the application fee. In fact, John had no business applying to any medical school in the United States, and he knew it. He went to Grenada instead, to St. George's, the medical school that was at the nexus of President Ronald Reagan's 1983 invasion of the island—where the lives of upward of 1,000 American medical students were at risk during Operation Urgent Fury.

John's description of *his* first day of medical school is as follows:

I remember the day I showed up in Grenada. I get off the airplane, and the airport is, you know, a single, open area. Hot as hell. Get off the plane and the humidity hits your face like a wall of sweat. And I remember there were some people there to greet us, from the university, and they put our bags in the van and we drove off to the... We drove around the countryside, and there's goats and chickens and people that are half-dressed. We go up and down and around roads [that] are all dusty, and all of a sudden the bus stops and the driver says, "We're here." And I'm looking around and I'm seeing dirt and rocks and goats and I'm thinking, "Where? Where are we? We're not here, where's here? There is no here. There's gotta be a here somewhere—let's go there."

No white-coat ceremony for John—way too hot for that.

The new Penn Med students weren't the only people on the stage who were in the process of a life transition. As it happened, this would be the last white-coat event for the medical school's highly respected dean, Dr. Arthur Rubenstein. He had announced his retirement a year earlier and wouldn't be there for the next one. This would be the last group of students to enter the school under his leadership, a period during which medical education had changed significantly. The new dean, Dr. Larry Jameson, would take his place the following year.

Rubenstein had seen the school through the evolution from a traditional four-year medical school curriculum, in which the first two years were spent in the classroom followed by two years of clinical work, to one in which a small-group paradigm, early exposure to patients and electronic learning have served as a national model. All medical school lectures are now filmed and available online; medical students no longer need to use microscopes or slides because the same material is presented on computer screens; and simulators are used to educate (in much the same way as in the airline industry)—to simulate surgery, cardiopulmonary resuscitation and trauma scenarios. The library, too, has changed. Where it was once stacked with medical texts old and new, and aisle after aisle of medical journals from all over the world, it has now gone digital; instead, there are rows upon rows of computer terminals.

Another change in the medical school curriculum speaks to what educators view as a major element of the future of medical care. Where medicine has traditionally been a field with a strong focus on the cult of the individual—the eminent pediatricians, internists and surgeons whose portraits and photos grace the walls of hospitals and medical schools all over the world—there is now an increasing emphasis on the importance of *teams* of professionals: doctors, nurses, pharmacists, and respiratory therapists working cohesively in the care of patients. Penn pioneered the introduction of the team theme into the curriculum; in fact, the team approach is embedded in the four-year medical education. Penn's 2010 entering class actually started medical school several days before its white-coat ceremony, with a two-day retreat including hula hoop, group movement and trust-building exercises (like falling back into the arms of others).

Team-building theory didn't originate in medicine, but its tenets are very applicable to complicated modern care. The exercises derive from the work of an educational psychologist named Bruce Tuckman, who coined terms for five stages of team evolution: forming, storming, norming, performing and adjourning. These processes encompass the activities typical of a group of individuals as they meet, sort out their roles and collaborate on how to complete some body of work before they actually start working. Penn Med's approach was designed in collaboration with its sister school, Penn's Wharton School of Business, which uses the same exercises and theories in its Graduate Leadership Program.

At both Wharton and Penn Med, students are randomly assigned to groups of six or seven on the first day of their retreat at an off-campus facility, and they start with team-building tasks in which there is no correct answer. In one example, two six-foot planks and some string were provided to six previously unacquainted students, with the assignment to cross a stretch of grass as a group, with no one touching a blade. While this may seem silly at first glance or inapplicable to medical care, it is not uncommon for a medical "code team" in a large hospital to consist of six individuals who don't know one another but are thrown together to work as a team in the middle of a high-stress patient-care crisis. Of course medical codes are typically *ad hoc,* one-off events, and the real intent of these exercises is to build a more durable group, analogous to that of a trauma or transplant team.

Tuckman's model was designed to build groups that accommodate the various talents that different individuals might bring to bear in a group activity—who's the leader, who are the problem solvers, who diffuses conflict—and to solve novel problems as they arise. One critical area for an effective team, for example, is to learn to disagree without letting it become personal—keeping it a "task conflict"—and move forward. Conflict of one sort or another is a daily event in every hospital, but there are constructive and destructive ways out.

It seems intuitive that we'd want physicians working collaboratively, but medicine has historically been a very autocratic field: the more senior the physician, the more dictatorial the mien. And surgical fields have traditionally been more militarily oriented than primary-care disciplines, perhaps because surgeons have been so integral to the care of wounded soldiers. The good intern follows her orders precisely, without *ever* complaining.

Earlier I mentioned Dr. Ravdin, the famous Penn and soldier surgeon. Legend has it that he intentionally stood on the foot of an intern throughout a lengthy operation, to see if the "kid" was made of the right stuff. The intern never complained and went on to become a prominent chair of surgery, years later. But while there's a certain romantic charm to the story, imagine the intern or nurse who, being a good soldier, or being too intimidated, doesn't speak up when some surgeon general of the operating room, perhaps with some traits of a tin-pot despot, starts to amputate the wrong breast of a woman with cancer.

Wrong-sided surgery has happened with fingers and toes, arms and legs, breasts, buttocks, eyes and ears and kidneys, testicles, lungs and brain lobes. There are enough sad, preventable stories of wrong-sided surgery in the annals of medicine to make you mistrust doctors forever. The solution, one that's now a newly mandated method of medical teamwork, is the presurgical "time out," based on a similar approach adopted much earlier by the airline industry after disasters in which the crew or copilot failed to confront an errant captain of the cockpit. Cockpit management is a system in which every member of the flight team is expected to speak up, even if it means breaking ranks, when they see a problem. The preflight and prelanding checklists are designed to methodically run through the aircraft settings prior to these critical portions of a flight.

The medical profession has begun to adopt schemes modeled on cockpit management and flight checklists. The preprocedural "time-out" is one of them. Before we begin a breast operation, for example, we follow a strict sequence of safety checks. Upon the patient's arrival in the preoperative area, one of the care team asks her which breast is being operated on. Her answer is verified with chart information, and the breast is marked by the surgeon with an indelible marker. And before the operation begins, one of the team—the circulating nurse, anesthesiologist or surgeon—stops everyone in the room and announces the name of the patient and the procedure to be performed. Once everyone has agreed, the first incision is made at the previously marked location.

Penn's students continue to work together in the same small team they were assigned to on day one throughout the first two years, in small humanism groups, while dissecting cadavers and while taking tests. And though it's not uncommon for individual members or splinter groups from these randomly assembled Penn Med or Wharton teams to ask for reassignment because they're unhappy with the chemistry, invariably they're told, "No, that's the whole point. Work it out." In effect the school's message is that "team" is part of the curriculum, that this is the new world order in medicine, and that while there may still be portraits for prominent practitioners and leaders, the new leaders will build and lead teams as a *part* of building their own careers.

John Pryor did so well at St. George's that he was able to transfer back to a U.S. medical school after two years. He entered the University at Buffalo, another New York state university. There he faced another branch point in his wandering career.

It came time to figure out what I wanted to do for a living. And that was not very easy at all. Again, I can't remember how much I was just thinking and how much I really felt because a lot of times in my life I'm not honest with myself. And I can't remember if I truly felt that I wanted to be a surgeon but I was doing medicine just because I wanted to cover all bases or if I truly couldn't think of being either medicine or surgery.

I do remember going back until I was in college, you know, feeling and looking at my hands and feeling that I should be a surgeon. Now that sounds really stupid. But I used to remember looking at my hands and saying, "These are hands of a surgeon."

I know that's stupid to say, but I knew, in my head, going backward—if you ask my parents they'll tell you my personality is definitely a surgical personality. But I didn't know what a surgical personality was when I was deciding between medicine and surgery.

John did go on to become a surgeon, a trauma surgeon in fact, which seemed to knit up many of the raveled threads of his life. As he narrates his story into the camera in that empty apartment with unshaven chin, he lets his hair down quite a long way.

I'm apprehensive about going to a new hospital because my big apprehension, my big fear, is meeting people and being embarrassed. I'm very self-conscious about what people think about me and what people say about me. It's always, I mean part of that is what drives me to be good and to be gracious and to be friendly, but part of it is the insecurity that probably goes back to when I was a kid and I wasn't totally accepted on the playground. I constantly worry about what people say about me. Now, I have to get over that because as soon as I get into a leadership role, running a trauma center, you can not be conscious of that anymore. You have to make decisions for the decision's merit and not worry about what people are going to say about ya. But there is a balance. There is a balance.

John never went through the team-building activity during medical school in Grenada, but he is exactly the kind of person Gail Morrison and the admissions team at the University of Pennsylvania would like to see entering medicine. He brought a well-rounded, experience-based perspective to his medical career—a perspective founded in his own life and his paramedical encounters with real patients as well as the books he had read in history and philosophy. John would eventually put this quotation from Albert Schweitzer—the great medical theologian, philosopher, musician and medical missionary—on the wall of his office:

Seek always to do some good, somewhere. Even if it's a little thing, do something for those who need help, something for which you get no pay but the privilege of doing it. For remember, you don't live in a world all your own. Your brothers are here, too.

John went on to complete a two-year fellowship in trauma and critical care at the University of Pennsylvania. By the end of that stretch he was so well liked and respected at Penn that he was asked to join the faculty.

Despite his insecurity and his apprehension, he led teams every day on rounds, at trauma alerts in the emergency room and in their care of severely injured patients in the operating room. But, unlike some faculty mentors of the past, John wasn't an autocrat; he was the epitome of a team player. He worried about the morale of the team. He took the feelings of every team member into account during stressful events, such as pulling the silently terrified medical student aside to reassure him in the midst of a trauma alert in which someone was dying from too many bullet wounds to count; or making sure the young nurse knew she hadn't done anything wrong during an operation in which she was a trainee scrub nurse; calmly teaching surgical residents and fellows as they encountered particularly difficult challenges during the maturation from novice to self-assured graduate.

John wasn't cast in the mold of I. S. Ravdin, the autocratic military surgeon. He was more like Nipper Schnabel, the compassionate internist. But he left indelible marks on everyone he trained, just as they did. John had just finished his training when the World Trade Center towers came down, and like many physicians, he headed immediately to New York on a train to help. And he was so moved by what he saw there that he enlisted in the Army and eventually ended up going to Iraq with a medical unit. He completed his tour there in 2006 with the 344th Combat Support Hospital.

After his return from service John wrote movingly of his experiences as a physician in opinion pieces in the *Philadelphia Inquirer* and the *Washington Post*, acknowledging the "palpable grief" the team felt when a soldier they'd cared for didn't survive.[9] He wrote of the hugs a military medical team exchanged after a death. There was no tin-pot dictator in John's ORs; there was a smoothly functioning, purpose-driven team, with all of its members pulling in the right direction, everyone feeling empowered.

John Pryor's approach to medical care and teaching is precisely what Arnold Gold was looking for when he formed his foundation to enhance humanism in medicine. Pryor's teams, which were often ad hoc collections of doctors and nurses, students and colleagues, exemplify the model that

Gail Morrison and the medical school faculty designed into the curriculum at Penn. With a lineage extending back to its founders—John Morgan, Edward Shippen and Ben Franklin—John and the rest of the faculty have evolved and adapted constantly as medicine and the world around it have changed.

As Gail Morrison puts it, regarding the integration of team-building activities into the medical school curriculum, "We're trying to make the next generation of physicians, and most of us believe that health care is going to be very much system driven. It's important to understand the difference between being a good team leader as opposed to being part of a group, and we're starting with this generation and saying 'this is what will make you different out there.'"

John Pryor redeployed to Iraq on December 9, 2008. He was very conflicted about leaving his wife, Carmela, a growing family, and colleagues who would consequently be one man short; but John felt that he had a duty to American military personnel as well. He ended up at a forward medical hospital in Mosul, Iraq. He continued to stay actively engaged with activities at Penn in the following weeks, mentoring the faculty member who had taken on his role as trauma director during his absence by providing real-time email advice. John liked email and sent several, often funny, lengthy messages every day. He was very attuned to new technologies and attentive to the ways in which they might change medical education and care in the future.

The concluding words in his 1999 video biography are:

So, that's it. Maybe in a couple of years we'll make another tape, kind of keep you updated. You've got all the other tapes. You know I'm using VCR technology and in 15 years from now, hopefully, we'll get all this digitalized to computer disk. If we're even using computer disks. Who the hell knows. Hopefully I'll be around to check in 15 years. So, see ya! In 2015.

On Christmas Day of 2008, I was sitting at the dinner table surrounded by my family in front of a comfortable fire when my cell phone rang. I remember we had all been laughing uproariously at some same oft-told family tale we trotted out every holiday. I'm not really sure what prompted me to answer it, but it seemed like an odd time for a call, so I thought it might be important. A good friend at the other end of the wire told me that John Pryor had been killed earlier that day during a mortar attack on the Mosul hospital facility in Iraq. He'd never made his daily call to his wife, and this was Christmas, so she knew something very bad had happened well before the two military officials arrived at her door.

It was only in the aftermath, when the shock had worn off, at memorial services and informal gatherings, that we all got a real sense of how widely John's influence had been felt. Everyone wanted to tell their own John Pryor story: his family, fellow faculty, friends, nurses, orderlies, medical students and military colleagues all had their own version of the way in which John had quietly propped them up personally at a bad moment, consoled the team after the death of a patient or dropped some funny, pithy pearl of wisdom into a terrible situation, defusing the tension and helping everyone get on about their work.

Great medical leaders of the past, like I. S. Ravdin, were sometimes feared even as they were admired and respected. And sometimes, with some leaders, that fear led to undesirable outcomes. John, on the other hand, was admired and beloved and had the ability to inspire his team members to do their best.

Research in many fields, including corporations, aviation and medicine, has shown that teams that work well together perform much better than those with a more top-down management style. Medical care in the future will be much more collaborative. John Pryor was posthumously promoted to the academic rank of associate professor. Despite, or perhaps because of, his meanderings on the way to a medical career, and maybe due to the absence of any semblance of arrogance, he became a perfect model for the kind of physician we'll need in the future.

CHAPTER 4

CODE!

Stanford University's medical school, like Penn's, now has a white-coat ceremony, and new students at both are handed the coat and a new stethoscope. But there's a difference. At the University of Pennsylvania, you get a coat, a stethoscope and a handshake from the dean. At Stanford, on the other hand, you get a coat, a stethoscope, a handshake *and* a brand new iPad, Apple's revolutionary "slate" computer. On August 23, 2010, the 91 new Stanford medical students were issued 32-gigabyte, Wi-Fi-enabled, touchscreen computers, loaded with virtual textbooks and equipped to wirelessly interface with the school's own online material as well as with a growing volume of remote online medical resources for medical professionals. And while the technical specs of this version of the device will soon become obsolete, Stanford's actions represent the dawn of a new era in medical education.

The cynical view could be that Apple and Stanford, Silicon Valley neighbors, have some product placement arrangement, evidenced by their students receiving complimentary copies of the most up-to-date gadgets. But the medical school had several explicit rationales, as described on its website[1]:

- Student readiness: Our students already have considerable familiarity and facility with educational technologies, and this creates new opportunities for efficient, mobile, and innovative learning.
- The flexibility of iPad technology: The iPad allows students to view and annotate course content electronically,

     facilitating advance preparation as well as in-class note-taking in a highly portable, sharable and searchable format.

- Access to information/Information Literacy: Students will be able to easily access high-quality information at any place, at any time (for example, images from textbooks on digital course reserve, image databases, journal articles, Lane Library's various search tools, etc.).
- "Going green": Replacing printed syllabi with PDF's [*sic*] is in line with the Sustainable Stanford initiative, which aims to build sustainable practices into every aspect of campus life.

Research into multiple intelligences has shown that there are many kinds of learners; some do better with visual data, and others with text. The Stanford students were oriented to the new devices with some directions from the school's instructional technology officer. "He addressed the students at a tutorial on how to use their iPads and pointed to a two-foot pile of binders. "This is the material for one course," he said. "We want to get you started going paperless. There's a lot less for you to carry around.... We want you to use the iPad when working with your cadavers in anatomy, or viewing slides in pathology, [although] no one has to use the iPad exclusively, or even at all."[2]

The new Stanford students have access to more than just portable technology. The school just opened a new medical education building, named after Chinese entrepreneur and philanthropist Li Ka Shing. Born into a poor family, Li Ka Shing never completed his own education in any traditional sense; he worked instead in a plastics factory in Hong Kong. But through hard work and shrewd investments, he eventually became one of the wealthiest men in the world. He sent his own son, Victor, to Stanford, and described their first visit to the Palo Alto campus: "As we walked together past these beautiful buildings, I was overtaken by everything this university represents and the opportunities it provides for students. On that occasion, I remember looking at Victor and saying, 'This is the first time in my life that I feel jealous.'"[3] Mr. Li's philanthropic investments have been varied but largely focused on education. In fact the new medical building is one of three Stanford projects he has supported.

The Li Ka Shing building is intended for use by students, residents, faculty and visitors and is one of the most advanced medical simulation centers

in the world. Its medical dummies, sophisticated $60,000–$90,000 mannequins, are comparable to flight simulators. In fact, these faux patients are so
sophisticated that they can be programmed to discharge too little urine, or
too much, and to tremble, sweat or bleed. Attached monitors may suggest
that they're suffering from a variety of diseases, including traumatic injuries, fluid in the lungs or high blood pressure. "The new center is also one
of the very few medical simulation centers in the world that brings together
many different types of mock-ups—using not just computerized dummies,
but also avatars and real actors."[4]

Simulation centers are increasingly common in medical schools around
the world. Medical simulation can be used to educate, test or stress students
or practicing professionals. The variety of approaches to the reproduction of
a medical scenario ranges from a simple on-screen computer program using
mouse and keyboard input to complicated scripts designed with humans,
mannequins and artificial intelligence. As with airline, nuclear power and
military simulation, there is a growing acknowledgement in medicine that
practitioners are better prepared if they've been through situations that
approximate real-life crises, and that, with the help of advances in technology, we are increasingly able to script scenarios that effectively duplicate
emergency room, operating room and intensive care disasters.

A "code blue" is typically the most stressful event in a young doctor's or
nurse's career. As a resident, I was called to respond to codes in the middle of
rounds, during meals, and when sleeping, going to the bathroom or shower-
ing. As I think back today, the stress, fatigue and sadness that I experienced
during some of these youthful encounters seem to have leached away; they
are lodged in the "adventures–experienced" section of my memories. But
in the intervening years I've also had to deliver a lot of bad news to families who were unprepared for it, and I've been through my own personal
losses that have unalterably changed the aura of codes and crises. Whatever
thrill I might have experienced during a code in the past is now gone; but
my experiences from residency are fairly typical and represent the medical
equivalents of war stories.

A nurse called me one night during residency when I was sleeping in a
call room in the basement of the Philadelphia veterans' hospital and yelled
"CODE!" into the phone before hanging up. But she didn't tell me where
the code was, and the hospital housed several hundred beds. Back then,
there was no caller ID, so I had no way of knowing where she'd called from.

I knew there was an emergency somewhere in the building and that I was responsible for a dying patient, but I didn't know where he was. Eventually, with some help from the nursing supervisor, I found out where I needed to be, but got there too late.

I was the designated code resident another day, a couple of years later. While my team was rounding in the intensive care unit of the Palo Alto veterans' hospital, which for some reason had a nine-hole golf course woven around its grounds, the operator announced over the public address system, "Code Blue on the golf green." Like the nurse in Philadelphia, however, she failed to say at which hole. We looked at each other, paused for a second, and then grabbed drugs, a defibrillator and IV equipment. We sprinted toward the nearest point on the course. Fortunately, we weren't too far off; there was a little cluster of people surrounding a downed middle-aged woman on the fourth green. Her husband stood next to her and was obviously distraught, holding his hands to his mouth.

The defibrillator was equipped with paddles that could display the patient's heart rhythm; the woman was in full cardiac arrest. We defibrillated a couple of times, inserted a breathing tube and intravenous lines—all while kneeling on the grass. The woman eventually converted to a normal rhythm. She was hospitalized, recovered from her cardiac arrest and pneumonia that complicated it and survived. Months later, she returned to the hospital to thank us. It turned out that she had an underlying cardiac abnormality that made her susceptible to abnormal heart rhythms, but it was easily treated with medication. This was a dramatic example of a code, one that even the most imaginative simulation designers might have struggled to come up with.

Another time, I was summoned early one morning by beeper to a code in a separate building as I emerged from the shower after a gritty night on call. Without bothering to towel-off completely, I pulled on some scrubs and lit out. Realizing that I had no shoes on as I headed up the stairs, I decided to continue without them. The nurses and doctors who were driving in to work would have seen me dashing across the lawn, half-dressed, like some crazy person from the psychiatric unit on the premises. Adding to the chaos, the automatic sprinkler system started up when I was about halfway to my destination, instantaneously converting the dash into more of a hurdle or steeplechase. I managed to clear a few sprinkler heads but eventually got sprayed. When I finally arrived at the indicated location, I was drenched in sweat and water, and chagrined to find that the call had been a false alarm.

Codes are ambushes: one minute you're at rest, or perhaps asleep, and the next, all hell breaks loose. You have to run to a place that is sometimes hard to find; once there, you have to make a rapid assessment of the scene—what's the problem, what are the possibilities, what's the data—and then act, often with incomplete information.

When I first became a faculty member, codes were, by tradition, directed by interns, the most-junior doctors on a medical team. I'm not sure how it came to be that way; perhaps it stemmed from a recognition that most in-hospital codes at that time wouldn't result in a good outcome anyway—the patient usually died. Or maybe it was merely a function of convenience; interns were typically the most readily available members of the team—they rarely showered, ate or slept while on duty.

I eventually became a member of the hospital Code Call Committee, and a few of us made the suggestion that we transfer responsibilities for codes to more-senior, seasoned residents who, presumably, had had more experience watching and participating in codes, not to mention more medical knowledge. After some deliberation, we decided to make the change. It helped. Codes became less chaotic.

It is easy to distinguish between a well-run code and more hectic ones by the number of people in play and the decibel level. In the former, there is a clear leader, and all team members know their roles. Someone at the head of the bed handles airway and breathing, usually an anesthesiologist or respiratory therapist. Someone else performs chest compressions; this can be physically demanding, so the compressor rotates out periodically. Still others may be working on IVs and measuring the patient's blood pressure, if there is any. A clerical person charts the data: vital signs, administered drugs and incoming labs. Well-run codes are quiet and businesslike, but all too often a lot of amped-up people start yelling, and order quickly descends into anarchy.

Codes make for good drama and often find their way into medical television scripts, but there are actually medical situations even *more* stressful than codes. These only occur in certain high-risk fields, and only to doctors of a certain age, with a certain degree of experience. One of these moments of crisis has that charged, silent feeling of the atmosphere before a severe electrical or wind storm, when the atmospheric pressure has plummeted. And sometimes that ominousness may only be evident to a single person in a crowded room.

The pulse oximeter is a cleverly designed medical instrument that measures how red, and therefore how well oxygenated, the blood is. A laser-like beam of light is sent through the bed of a patient's nail and is measured on the other side and the wavelength of the measured light correlates with the blood's color. The oximeter was designed for use by anesthesiologists in the operating room. Prior to this invention, the only way you'd know if a patient was getting into trouble during surgery was if the skin turned blue. The "pulse ox" converted a very subjective measure to a very precise one—one that works equally well with light- and dark-skinned patients.

The designers of this sensitive instrument did something else very clever. Just as with traditional EKGs, the oximeter beeps with each heartbeat, so the anesthesiologist and surgeon can tell without looking whether the heart is beating faster or slower—either of which can indicate a problem. But unlike the EKG, the beep of each heartbeat on the pulse ox changes in pitch, depending on the amount of oxygen in the blood, so the trained doctor can listen for two critical pieces of information without ever looking up at a screen. A quickening heart rate going up with a steady, unchanging high pitch may mean that the patient is waking up, while a slowing heart rate with a pitch that descends from a steady *beep, beep, beep*, to a *beop…beop…beop*, and thence to a *booop……. boooop……* means something altogether different— not enough oxygen in the patient's system.

As anesthesiologists, one of the first things we do after a patient is asleep is to insert a breathing tube, because controlling the airway is a critical part of our job. Most of the time, this is a routine process, but occasionally it's clear ahead of time that there is the potential for trouble, because a patient has physical characteristics like an underbite or obesity that correlate with airway anatomy trouble. There are ways to plan for these situations, but occasionally someone looks normal, who isn't. So you're caught flatfooted.

In one such situation, I was the anesthesiologist in the case of a teenage girl with an inflamed appendix. She needed an operation under general anesthesia to remove the diseased organ. We'd chatted while I gathered medical information, and then I rolled her litter into the operating room. She was very nervous, so I quickly inserted an IV and then injected Pentothal, a drug we use to put patients to sleep. I added a curare-like drug to paralyze the muscles of her tongue and jaw so that she wouldn't bite or gag when I inserted a breathing tube into her lungs. This use of a chemical relaxant, or paralytic, is routine, but these drugs also paralyze the breathing muscles, which meant that my patient could no longer breathe on her own—even if she was running out of oxygen. Again, this is usually routine; the anesthesiologist takes over the breathing, using a mask and bag to blow air in and out of the nose and mouth. But this time, unexpectedly, I couldn't insert the tube. She had a difficult airway.

Despite my squeezing of the bag, I couldn't blow any oxygen into her lungs because there was something blocking the airflow. There are many potential causes but not a lot of time to sort out the problem. There were other people in the room. The surgeon was talking to a couple of nurses in a corner, waiting to scrub his hands with a disinfectant. They were, at first, completely oblivious to my problem. Alone in this crisis, I tried different maneuvers unsuccessfully and could hear her heart rate increasing—60, then 70, then 90. At first, the pitch of the pulse oximeter fortunately stayed high. There was still enough oxygen in her bloodstream that critical organs like her heart and brain were still adequately supplied. But oxygen comes into the body through the airways, and they were blocked at this point. The others chatted away, but I could feel a charged silence quickly building up in the room, and I could smell the anesthetic leaking from around the edges of the mask because it wasn't getting into her lungs, where it needed to be.

At that instant I *knew*—and, of the folks in the room, only *I* knew—that if I didn't do the right thing in the next few seconds, this girl was going to die. Surgeons, too, have these crisis moments when they cut into a big blood vessel in an unexpected or difficult location. An experienced cardiologist may see the heart stop on the EKG even as a patient natters on for a last few seconds before his eyes roll back in his head. These brief intervals of impending doom are specific to certain high-risk medical fields. It's like the pilot who feels an unexpected shudder in the plane when birds hit the engines, or the marine walking "point" who spots an odd-looking piece of garbage while on foot patrol just before he sees the wire attached to it. These about-to-happen crises differ from medical codes where the die has effectively *already* been cast. During these terrifying, telescoping seconds, the wrong action, or even the right action taken too slowly, can end a life. The way one performs at those moments, and the way one handles the outcome once it's over, good or bad, can change a person forever.

When the pitch of the pulse oximeter first changed from a *high-C*, then to *B* and *B-flat*, and my patient's heart rate began to slow, I knew we only had seconds before brain damage became a real risk. I told the surgeon and nurses to "get a trach set" in that terse, clipped tone that signals unequivocally that "we have a crisis." The nurses ran to get the emergency tray of sterile equipment we've set aside for just this kind of situation and opened it. The surgeon quickly scrubbed his hands and put on a sterile gown and gloves. I poured an iodine solution on my patient's neck neck to prep the skin, and we put drapes around the base of the neck to frame out the area where we needed to insert the tracheostomy tube—the breathing tube that goes directly through front of the neck into the airway.

The surgeon made a quick, deep cut with the scalpel while the nurse suctioned away the blood that welled up. They cauterized the bleeding vessels and made a hole in the trachea (the windpipe). The surgeon inserted the tracheostomy tube, and I hooked up the oxygen circuit. It gave her a couple of big breaths full of oxygen, and, just as suddenly as it occurred, the crisis was over. The pulse oximeter's tone ran back up the scale, and her heart rate slowed. We proceeded with the operation and she woke up with no awareness of what had happened while she was asleep. We were able to remove the tracheostomy tube without problem during her short, subsequent hospitalization. My patient came away from the experience with only a small scar at the base of her throat.

When it happened, I was not expecting problems with this girl's airway, but *we* were prepared as a team. We had a trach set ready for just this unusual eventuality. And with the help of simulation training, we will do a much better job of preparing the next generation of medical professionals for routine and unusual problems and crises, using mock scenarios where a real patient is not at risk.

There's an old medical adage that speaks to the way medical procedures used to be taught. It goes like this: "See one. Do one. Teach one." It's catchy and is a pretty accurate description of the way we all used to learn back before we had simulators. Take the simple but extremely important act of placing a catheter in a vein.

As those of you know who've been through blood drawing or the insertion of an IV, some medical practitioners are very slick at doing this, but many aren't. I've had my own blood drawn inexpertly, and I remember leaving some of my patients punctured and bruised as a medical student. I only later progressed to a certain degree of competence. I particularly recall one kind, elderly lady who needed an IV but had extremely wiggly, fragile veins. She patiently and painfully lay there for over an hour as I tried repeatedly to get a catheter into a vein. Despite tears in her eyes, she kept saying, "It's all right, dear. I know you're trying." By the time I was done—after I did finally get a tiny catheter in a finger vein—both of her arms and one foot were bleeding from several sites. Many patients are much less gracious. And it is far worse with children, who have no idea why you are hurting them, sometimes over and over.

There are now simulators for IV placement and arterial line placement; dummy abdomens for laparoscopic surgical simulation; and entire trauma, emergency room, operating room or intensive care unit simulation suites— all of which can be designed to test the performance of both individuals and teams. It is even possible to create mass-casualty scenarios. Some simulations are run from a local control room. Others use network connections and remote, off-site trainers.

Basic and Advanced Cardiac Life Support is a curriculum designed to educate students about how to evaluate a patient suspected of having a life-threatening respiratory or cardiac problem in a code. During my training, we used dummy plastic heads and torsos and performed mock codes. The standard mannequin of the era was called *Resusci Anne*, although she lacked feminine features or parts. It was probably better that way, because we had to practice mouth-to-mouth resuscitation and chest compressions on Annie during the mock code test. Annie was an athlete, too. She always wore a track suit, which was easy to slip off when it came time to bare her chest for compressions or to get good contact between the defibrillator paddles and her bosom.

The Resusci Anne product is marketed by a Norwegian company, founded in the 1940s, called Laerdal, which originally marketed toys. The mannequin's face has a lifelike quality, and there's an interesting story behind that face. It is actually based on that of a real woman—a young girl, as it turns out—who was found drowned in Paris's River Seine in the late 1800s. As was the custom of the era, when photography was not widely available, a death mask was made of her features for potential later identification. There was no evidence of violence on the body, and it was rumored that she was a suicide, possibly the victim of unrequited romance. Today, the bust of the Girl from the River Seine is featured on Laerdal's promotional materials. She has a delicate, almost-Grecian beauty.

Perhaps motivated by the war that broke out in the 1940s, Asmund Laerdal eventually steered his company away from toys and toward doll-like mannequins that could be used in wound and resuscitation training. But Laerdal also had direct personal experience with the effectiveness of resuscitation. His own son Tore nearly drowned as a two-year-old, and it was Asmund himself who cleared his child's airway and saved his life.[5] He came to believe that students would be stimulated to learn lifesaving cardiopulmonary resuscitation if the "victim" was life-sized and lifelike—hence the choice of Resusci Anne.

One had to perform a ritualized series of actions during mock codes in the 1980s to pass the certification exam. First you were to approach her, shouting, "Annie! Annie! Are you okay?" This typically got some laughs from the rest of the class the first few times. If Annie failed to awaken, and she always did, you were then required to yell loudly for help; "Look, Listen and Feel" for a breath; and then begin a series of mouth-to-mouth breaths and sternal (breastbone) compressions. Basic life support was the first emergency curriculum to evolve, but there are now similar programs in trauma, pediatrics and critical care. While each of these courses has its own textbook, and the material is continuously updated as the field advances, a core component usually revolves around skills stations, where one learns to do the specific procedures (like airway management) employed in life support, and simulated crises that have become increasingly realistic.

Over the years, Resusci Anne's descendants have become more and more lifelike. And Annie eventually found a mate: the sophisticated SimMan whose "durable and rugged construction provides you with the flexibility to perform simulation-based education in the environment of your choice. Built with the quality you've come to expect from Laerdal, SimMan 3G was developed to be the most reliable patient simulator in the world—giving you the peace of mind to know that you can train where you practice medicine—in real environments with real results."[6] SimMan's embedded microsensors measure how well a trainee is performing compressions. He can be programmed to develop a whole sequence of lethal arrhythmias, and he has fake veins. Annie and SimMan even took some family leave to make a baby, SimNewB, equipped with a lifelike umbilical cord and the ability to cry and move. SimNewB can even play dead, turning a dusky blue and losing his simulated heartbeat.

Laerdal now markets an entire suite of mannequins, simulation control equipment and courses designed to educate medical professionals and laypersons in the skills required to save a life. There's even a line of Laerdal face shields on key rings. The shield is intended to cover a victim's face and mouth, still permitting a rescuer to administer mouth-to-mouth breaths but preventing contamination from secretions. The face shield pouches come in red, green, blue, yellow, black and camouflage and can be silk-screened with a company's logo.

At Stanford's Immersive Learning Center, its *virtual theater* is capable of showing life-sized, three-dimensional images of the human body and its parts. Technologies that originated in the motion-picture industry and were designed for immersive fantasy (as in the movie *Avatar*), are being embraced by pioneers in medical education. Stanford's skills-training suite has mechanical and virtual trainers to teach specific skills. And the procedures and scenarios aren't attempted just once; they are drilled over and over again until the trainee demonstrates a satisfactory level of competence before becoming certified to "Do One" on a real patient.

Stanford's simulation center isn't just a shell with a brain. It is a smart building: video cameras throughout can capture audiovisual material for an archive, for simultaneous remote viewing by a larger audience elsewhere in the building or for presentation on the web. Operating theaters of the past had amphitheaters surrounding the operating table, as in Thomas Eakins's great surgical portraits of the Agnew and Gross Clinics. Later, trainees watched surgery from balconies over the operating table in medical television dramas like Drs. Casey, Welby and Kildare. Today's procedures are broadcast live to remote theaters—warts and all—from a "surgeon's-eye view," using head-mounted cameras and mikes as audiovisual feeds.

The Li Ka Shing center has more technology than most of the other buildings on the Stanford campus, including nine million dollars' worth of audiovisual equipment. But the smart teaching technologies on display at this brand new educational center will soon be eclipsed at hospitals that are deploying smart patient rooms and buildings around the country.

The University of Pittsburgh has partnered with IBM in designing a suite of software and hardware intended to organize and facilitate the interactions of doctors, nurses and patients. The room "recognizes" a provider when she enters a room by her ultrasonic identification badge, automatically presents relevant information from the electronic medical record and responds to voice commands. The room "reminds" providers to wash their hands by illuminating the hand-washing station. It can also distinguish among different types of hospital personnel and display one set of information to a dietary worker, another to the phlebotomist before he draws blood and more detailed information to doctors and nurses. The UPMC SmartRoom is intended to leverage the information contained in electronic health records and deliver it to the right provider, about the right patient, at the right time.

General Electric has gone quite a bit further in their smart-medical room design. The GE room uses optical sensors, radio frequency identification (RFID) tags, facial recognition, computer-vision algorithms, cameras and speakers that are subtly deployed throughout the room. The software is designed to track the activities of health-care workers and patients for different reasons. By identifying individual workers and monitoring their compliance with best practices, such as hand-washing, the system can be used to continuously improve performance. The smart room can also track patients' movements to determine whether they are, for example, out of bed without assistance and therefore at risk for a fall, or moving erratically, indicating a possibly developing delirium. GE believes we may even eventually be able to identify facial expressions characteristic of an evolving stroke or severe pain by using computer-vision algorithms.[7]

The integration of highly precise, miniaturized sensors with ubiquitous wireless communications and computing systems will undoubtedly lead to dramatic changes in the way we practice and experience medical care, in both the hospital and the home.

CHAPTER 5

STRETCH, FLOSS, DANCE AND MENTOR

The University of Pennsylvania's campus is typical of Ivy League schools and many other great old universities of the world. Old buildings with greenery crawling up the walls. Statues of historic figures. And avant-garde sculptures plunked hither and yon. The commons has a larger-than-life figure of Ben Franklin sitting in a chair atop a giant pedestal; Claes Oldenburg's giant work called *The Split Button* seems to have been dropped on the plaza in front of the library; and a copy of the *LOVE* statue, designed by Robert Indiana for this country's bicentennial, sits on a little rise at the top. Walkways crisscross the space, which has a significant slope. Skateboarders are discouraged by the campus police but invariably return quickly after having been shooed away. But no one hassles Dr. Stephen Gluckman when he whisks by on his fold-up scooter.

Steve has a medical practice located several blocks away from the hospital, and he often has to move quickly from one location to the other. While many of our colleagues have this same problem, most of them take the shuttle bus. Steve likes the exercise and the freedom of the scooter. Wearing the long white coat of a full-faculty member, with its tails flapping in the breeze, he weaves deftly in and out through crowds of students. He's short and trim, has a full beard and the erect posture of a habitual exerciser; and he cuts a striking figure as he crosses the green under the watchful eyes of old Ben on his perch. He's well into his sixties, but looks no older than 50. His eyes are shrewd and twinkle behind his glasses.

Steve Gluckman is an infectious disease specialist and an expert in tropical diseases. While the tropical diseases I learned about in school 30 years ago were malaria and parasites, today's most prevalent problems in many tropical and third-world countries are tuberculosis and HIV/AIDS. Steve has seen a lot of both, having helped in Botswana to direct a growing medical program, the product of a partnership between Penn's medical school and both the Republic and the University of Botswana. The collaboration started in 2001, prompted by the country's HIV/AIDS crisis. It initially began when the African Comprehensive HIV/AIDS Partnership—a collaboration of the Gates Foundation, the Merck Foundation and the country of Botswana—solicited help from Penn's HIV experts, including Gluckman.

The prevalence of HIV/AIDS in adults in Botswana is estimated to be 24 percent, one of the highest of any nation in the world (second only to Swaziland). Yet the country is economically stable, due in part to income from its diamond mines, and has a robust health-care system. The Penn/Botswana program has made dramatic improvements in the distribution of antiretroviral drugs to patients with the disease and has started public health campaigns using slogans like: "Abstinence, Be Faithful and Condomize," the ABCs of AIDS. But, as Gluckman put it to me one day when we were sitting in his office and speaking about the medical students who were headed to Botswana for training: "One of the things they're going to see, *guaranteed*, every day is people dying of things there that they won't die of here."

Another Penn faculty member, Dr. Jason Kessler, described his own wake-up call in Penn's alumni publication, the *Gazette*[1]:

> "One of my earliest experiences here in Botswana that stands out in my mind involved a young man in his early twenties. He was admitted to the hospital with signs of meningoencephalitis (infection of the brain and its surrounding tissues) and was begun on antibiotics for a presumed bacterial infection.
>
> "This unfortunate young man was delirious, feverish, and his family had brought him to the hospital after his condition continued to deteriorate at home," Kessler recalls. He was also found to be HIV-positive, though it was not clear whether the two conditions were linked.

After seeming to stabilize over the next day or so, the patient fell unconscious. "We tried desperately to initiate the measures I was used to as a trainee in the U.S.—paging doctors, starting IVs, resuscitation—but as we continued our efforts, which seemed to be getting nowhere, the patient began groaning," Kessler says. "Loud, awful groans that reverberated through the ward, causing all the families in the area to turn and watch us as we struggled. It wasn't more than a minute or so later that the patient arrested and died in front of us all.

"The suddenness and the fierceness of death stunned and shocked me," he says. "I don't think I had really witnessed anyone, especially someone so young, die in my presence. Of course, I had been present at 'codes' during residency but that experience was more similar to a drill—a bunch of people in a room carrying out different tasks in a generally organized fashion. The patient (in those codes) seemed almost irrelevant and completely dehumanized. This was something so completely different and disturbing. It opened my eyes to the nature of illness here—people my age or even younger dying every day, and my limits as a doctor to help many of them."

Penn now sends nurses, students, residents and faculty to Botswana throughout the year, and the partnership has expanded to include a broad range of medical disciplines. Dermatologists, working with Botswana's doctors, provide telemedical consultations when needed. Dr. Carrie Kovarik, an expert on tropical dermatological diseases, leads an effort in which providers in Africa fill out a computerized form and send accompanying cell-phone photographs of a patient's skin lesions to Penn, where they're evaluated by an expert.

Penn has also been experimenting with text messaging to improve care, working with a private medical practice in Botswana to see if cell-phone text-message reminders improve the rate at which HIV patients refill prescriptions, visit physicians and reduce their viral loads. If successful, the technology would help address the country's current shortage of doctors and nurses, freeing up medical workers to concentrate on the sickest patients. Similar programs have been used elsewhere for other diseases, like malaria. There are also nascent efforts to begin a streamlined electronic medical record for African patients, so that each new visit will begin with some baseline information from past visits.

Steve Gluckman was one of an initial group of Penn doctors who traveled to Botswana in reply to their initial request for help in 2001. He played a key role in the growth of the relationship, serving as the clinical director of the program for almost ten years. For a while, he practiced medicine in Africa for almost five months a year. He spent his time there caring for patients who lay on mattresses in overcrowded wards, with young people dying of diseases that would be easily treatable elsewhere. And then he'd return to Penn, to the technology-rich intensive care unit where I practice, to serve as an academic, Western infectious disease specialist.

In the Penn ICU he would consult on cases of gangbangers with gunshot injuries and octogenarians who'd spent the last several months of their lives on ventilators and dialysis. He'd watch us burn through expensive supplies that are used once and then discarded, where the same equipment would be used repeatedly or would be unavailable in Botswana. Then he'd return to Africa and to the young African victims of the AIDS epidemic and untreated rheumatic fever. We've talked about this a number of times, and the contrasts between the two worlds clearly trouble him. He has had a unique vantage point as he has shuttled back and forth between two starkly different medical realities, accumulating a store of pearls of wisdom that apply equally well to the practice of medicine in both worlds.

Despite his perambulations, and his resulting intermittent availability, Steve is regarded as a doctor's doctor, the kind of physician to whom other physicians entrust themselves for care and advice. He's also revered as a teacher and humanist by medical students, residents and fellows in both worlds. One of the common features of white-coat ceremonies in medical, nursing and pharmacy schools is a keynote address to the students by a respected clinician who epitomizes the humanistic values celebrated at these events. It wasn't surprising to anyone that Dr. Gluckman was selected as the keynote speaker for the University of Pennsylvania's 2010 white-coat ritual that I described earlier.

I arrived late to the ceremony and missed the live version of his remarks, but I caught a recorded version later on the school's website. Like all of the medical school's lectures, it was taped and could be streamed on demand. Steve's speech was unpretentious but profound. It wasn't about lofty ambitions or ideals. It was more like the now infamous 1997 "Wear Sunscreen" recommendations often attributed to a commencement address by Kurt Vonnegut but was actually written as a *Chicago Tribune* column by Mary

Schmich.[2] Her discourse actually begins, "Inside every adult lurks a gradua-tion speaker dying to get out, some world-weary pundit eager to pontificate on life to young people who'd rather be rollerblading. Most of us, alas, will never be invited to sow our words of wisdom among an audience of caps and gowns, but there's no reason we can't entertain ourselves by composing a Guide to Life for Graduates."[3] The column is more formally titled: "Advice, Like Youth, Probably Just Wasted on the Young." Like Gluckman, Schmich bases her counsel on her own "meandering experiences."

All in all, by the end of his white-coat keynote address to the medi-cal students, Steve made 12 recommendations, 11 of which relate to being a doctor, and the last of which speaks to remaining human on the job. His first piece of advice was: "Develop trust in your clinical skills."[4] Like Mary Schmich's admonitions to "wear sunscreen" and "floss," this is deceptively simple advice. Young people tend not to look after their skin or teeth the same way older ones do; they take the short view. Similarly, today's young clinicians tend neither to look at their patients nor to trust in their still-to-be-honed skills of observation; they test rather than touch. This, too, is shortsighted.

The best doctors of every generation from Hippocrates to the present are the ones who look, listen and feel their way to a sense of confidence in their clinical skills. Dr. Joseph Bell was one of these. A nineteenth-century lec-turer at the University of Edinburgh, Bell was very good at looking, listening and feeling for information about his patients. He was said to have walked with a jerky kind of a step that communicated great energy and athleticism. His nose and chin were angular. And his eyes twinkled with shrewdness. In addition to being a brilliant doctor, Dr. Bell was also an amateur poet and a bird-watcher.

Dr. Bell watched the way a person moved. He had noted that the walk of a sailor varied vastly from that of a soldier. If he identified a person as a sailor, he would then look for tattoos that might tell where that sailor had been. He trained himself to listen for small differences in his patients' accents to help him identify where they came from. Bell studied and felt the hands of his patients because calluses or other marks could help him determine their occupation.

"In teaching the treatment of disease and accident," Dr. Bell said, "all careful teachers have first to show the student how to recognize accurately the case. The recognition depends in great measure on the accurate and rapid appreciation of small points in which the diseased differs from the healthy state. In fact, the student must be taught to observe. To interest him in this kind of work we teachers find it useful to show the student how much a trained use of the observation can discover in ordinary matters such as the previous history, nationality and occupation of a patient."[5]

Bell served as Queen Victoria's personal surgeon when she visited Scotland. He became a fellow of the Royal College of Surgeons of Edinburgh. He died in 1911 at the age of 74, but not before he'd inspired the development of one of the greatest fictional characters in all of literature. Arthur Conan Doyle, the author of the Sherlock Holmes stories, served as Bell's assistant in his clinic and modeled the famed detective on his mentor. Bell developed his almost supernatural skills of observation in his practice as a physician, and it is rumored that he identified Jack the Ripper in a letter he mailed to Scotland Yard. The murders perpetrated by the serial killer ceased immediately thereafter.[6]

Like Joseph Bell, Steve Gluckman's advice to the newly minted medical students to trust in their clinical skills comes from years spent in hospitals where the most accurate tool is often the stethoscope. Many of today's new trainees feel more comfortable ordering a CT scan to diagnose pneumonia, when equally accurate information could be gathered by looking at and listening to the patient's chest and lungs.

"Be compulsive." This was Steve's second suggestion. We order lots of tests in modern hospitals, but we occasionally fail to check the results. I have a physician friend who, at a time early in his career, ordered a lab test on a patient but failed to look up the results himself or to assign the responsibility to another before he left at the end of his shift. The patient was dead by the time he arrived the next morning. Had he checked, he would have found that the patient had a critically low potassium level—something that could have been very simply corrected in a matter of minutes. We put lots of checks and balances in place to prevent this kind of thing; however, almost invariably a series of errors line up like holes in Swiss cheese when unexpected deaths occur. My friend has had to live with the guilt of that omission and its grave consequences ever since. "Be compulsive."

In an earlier chapter, I mentioned that moment when I needed to call for the tracheostomy set as I struggled to get air into a young patient's lungs. At the time, my need to call for help felt like an admission of failure; but it was at an early point in my career—I know better now. Steve's third piece of advice is: "Ask for help." Like Steve, I've come to believe that one of the most telling signs of immaturity in a medical trainee—a resident or fellow—is an unwillingness to seek advice or help when needed. A call for help may take the form of a generalist asking a specialist for consultation on an obscure disease, or it may be a less-experienced physician running an unusual situation by a respected elder. Sometimes someone who's just too tired, perhaps after an all-night operation, asks for help from a fresher set of hands. A good doctor knows when to ask for help.

Most young doctors have been extremely successful in most of what they've done and are often attracted to the field of medicine because its practitioners are typically self-confident, competent people. But there is a fine line in medicine between competence and self-confidence on the one hand, and overconfidence and arrogance on the other. The godlike archetype of the doctor of yore has come into disfavor as we increasingly recognize that teams of providers function more effectively than any single individual who may be loath to ask for assistance when needed or fails to recognize his own fallibilities.

The fourth thing Steve told the incoming medical students at the white-coat ceremony was: "Be honest with your patients." There's a legal and ethical doctrine in medicine known as *informed consent*. Today's patients are asked to sign all sorts of informed consent documents for hospital admission, research protocols, blood transfusions, surgical procedures and anesthesia, among others. These documents serve as legal protection and are designed to trigger a conversation between the provider and the patient in which several key elements are discussed: the nature of the decision or procedure; reasonable alternatives to the proposed intervention; relevant risks, benefits and uncertainties related to each alternative; an assessment of patient understanding; and, finally, the acceptance of the intervention by the patient.

The concept of informed consent arose as a consequence of the sadistic medical experiments performed on non-consenting experimental subjects by the Nazis during World War II. The doctrine was formally described in the Nuremberg Code when it was adopted in 1948.[7] But Steve Gluckman's counsel to "be honest" is about more than just the procedural requirements of consent; it's about the establishment of trust and truth between doctor and patient.

A good doctor has to ask difficult questions of her patients. Do they hurt? Do they smoke, drink or take drugs? How is their sex life? Do they use condoms or birth control? Do they pass blood in their urine or stool? There's a lot of room for misinterpretation when these conversations aren't handled tactfully.

Patients have lots of fears that they may hide or that may seem ridiculous and unfounded to a busy medical professional. Imagine the patient who's just read of a celebrity's death from anal cancer and then notices blood in the toilet after his own bowel movement. It's embarrassing and scary and can be difficult to talk about for both reasons. To the doctor, however, the hemorrhoids she may find on exam are a trivial, routine problem. Or she may find cancer, just as her patient feared. These are two very different conversations. An honest relationship between the doctor and the patient is at the very foundation of the profession. This admonition to be honest and the rest of Steve's pearls of medical wisdom are essential for young doctors as they begin their training.

"Take responsibility for being someone's doctor." The growing recognition of the importance of teamwork in medical care shouldn't be allowed to diminish the importance of a one-to-one relationship between a provider and his patient. I sit on a committee at my hospital where we see the letters of complaints from patients about their medical care. To be sure, the vast majority of the letters we get are complimentary; but a small group of doctors get more than their share of complaints. The odd thing is that some of these doctors are internationally respected and get referrals from all over the country.

The problem in many cases is that they've become, or, in some cases, perhaps they've always been, technicians—extremely skilled at what they do, but technicians nonetheless. Often these doctors have become so busy that they're always in the operating room or traveling extensively to talk about their work. Some of them were never very good with people to begin with, but they're very good at research. Whatever the case, they generate complaints, often even when providing good care. They have a low social IQ.

The fundamental problem in almost every instance is that they weren't following that most critical piece of Steve's advice: "Take responsibility for being someone's doctor." This means talking to your patient honestly about the risks and benefits of a treatment, seeing it through and being there at the far end regardless of whether or not the results were favorable. As medicine has become more and more complex, and there are more handoffs from one provider to another, it's become very easy for providers to hide behind the system. But they mustn't.

Good doctors loop back over and over again to check on their patients. They take ownership—and keep it, even after handing off an issue to a consultant. This is a fundamental premise of the "patient-centered medical home," a topic I'll elaborate on later. Mary Schmich says, "Don't be reckless with other people's hearts." And by saying "be honest," and "take responsibility," Steve Gluckman is telling the incoming medical school class: "Don't be reckless with other people's trust." Good doctors aren't.

While most of these extremely talented young people don't need to hear it, his sixth recommendation was: "Set high standards for yourself." He's saying, "Don't do sloppy work, don't keep sloppy records, don't sew sloppy stitches that leave scars, don't leave a mess for another to clean up, and don't assign someone else to deliver bad news." Good doctors are hard on themselves—not self-destructive, mind you—but they're not complacent or satisfied with "just good enough."

The counterpoint to being hard on yourself is Steve's next admonition: "Be forgiving of yourself." It is possible to be too soft on oneself—to have low standards—or to be too ambitious—to set inappropriately or unachievably high goals. A physician should not aspire to godlike perfection. Medicine is a human undertaking, one that may have evolved from the simple act of grooming among primates. The very best doctors question their performance constantly—"Was there a better way to handle that?"—without destroying themselves in the process. Mary Schmich's way of thinking about this is: "Maybe you'll marry, maybe you won't. Maybe you'll have children, maybe you won't. Maybe you'll divorce at 40, maybe you'll dance the funky chicken on your 75th wedding anniversary. Whatever you do, don't congratulate yourself too much, or berate yourself either. Your choices are half chance. So are everybody else's."

Proof of continuing medical education in the form of CME credits is increasingly required for ongoing licensure in many countries. These credits can be acquired by attendance at conferences, online educational activities and teaching. CME requirements are designed to codify Steve Gluckman's eighth adjuration: "Develop lifelong learning habits."

Medical information is constantly being rewritten. Genomics, stem-cell therapies and nanomedicine have all developed during my 30-year professional career, as have laparoscopy, robotic surgery and new forms of radiation like stereotactic radiosurgery and proton therapy. New specialties and sub-specialties develop every year. Medicine is a giant ecosystem that's in constant ferment. Physicians who fail to stay current, to read and to evolve get left by the wayside, which is a problem for their patients and a missed opportunity for themselves.

Mary Schmich has lots of sound life advice that speaks to the joys of lifelong learning: "Do one thing every day that scares you," she says. In other words, don't ever get in a comfort zone. Stay edgy. "Sing" and "Stretch" and "Don't feel guilty if you don't know what you want to do with your life. The most interesting people I know didn't know at 22 what they wanted to do with their lives. Some of the most interesting 40-year-olds I know still don't."

Stay interested. Develop lifelong learning habits. Adopt an attitude of inquisitiveness rather than authority. The greatest medical teachers I know are the ones who say, "I don't know" when they don't; "That's a really good question" when it is; and, "Let's look that up."

It used to be hard to look it up, though. The answers to questions might or might not be in a medical library, and, while the library was usually open late, it might be locked when that really odd question came up in the middle of the night. Today, we're really lucky. The library is open all night, it's enormous, the Dewey Decimal system has been replaced by hyperlinks and search engines, and it's all available on our smartphones.

Steve's ninth command is: "Don't go to bed with clinical questions left on your mind from the day's work." But now I can get into my bedclothes, fire up the iPad or my cell phone, and browse *my* library or someone else's, the medical literature or a host of disease-specific websites—or even pose a question on a listserv to colleagues across the world—all from the comfort of my own bed. Steve is saying, "Stay hungry for knowledge," and "Don't go to bed un-sated."

Schmich advises: "Enjoy your body. Use it every way you can. Don't be afraid of it or of what other people think of it. It's the greatest instrument you'll ever own," and "Read the directions, even if you don't follow them." Great doctors enjoy their *minds* and use them every way they can. They revel in the ever-changing landscape of the field. While they read the directions about taking care of humans in medical journals and texts, they also understand that those instructions are only written in pencil—that medical research is constantly revealing new sets of directions.

Steve's final two suggestions about how to become a good doctor are about teaching and mentoring, two different but related activities. In a sense, he's doing both in giving the keynote address. He says: "Teach at every opportunity," and "Mentor." When he first arrived in Botswana, the mission of the Penn HIV/AIDS specialists was to help the country get a handle on the growing epidemic. As he described it,

> There wasn't any concept at the time that Penn's involvement would be ongoing.... It was meeting after meeting, and sort of boring. So I asked, "Where is the local hospital?" They pointed me to Princess Marina, and I went over there and sat in a couple of conferences and asked if I could do rounds with them. That was a three-month stint, and by the end of it, I had my own [medical] service.
>
> When we got there, there was no teaching in the hospital at all.... There was no signing out when people left, no handing off of patients, and essentially no coverage [by doctors] on the weekends.... Most doctors there are just hired by the government and they have a contract to work.... There is nothing in their contracts that says they have to care, or to read about medicine, and it has taken a fair amount [of effort] to get them to buy into why all that stuff is good. [But] they *have* bought into it, and that's been really gratifying—in many ways more so than the individual patient encounters.[8]

Steve is a consummate teacher. He teaches patients how to care for themselves and medical students how to care for patients. He's mentored countless young doctors in their ongoing careers. His teaching and mentoring—as well as that of other faculty from the medical, nursing, communications and business schools—have evolved into a growing collaboration between the University of Pennsylvania and the University of Botswana. The two schools have recently partnered in the development of the country's first medical school.

When I'm asked what I do at social gatherings or my kid's athletic events, I answer that I'm a doctor, which is usually followed by questions about what kind and where do I practice. When I answer that I'm on the faculty at the University of Pennsylvania, some people want to know if I teach. When I say yes, they want to know if I do so in a classroom. While I have done some classroom teaching, I don't any more. But I do teach every time I take care of a patient, because that's the way we practice at a university hospital. We practice and teach at the same time. Whether it's during rounds on patient wards, at an operating room table or while reading films in the radiology viewing room, we're always working side by side with residents and medical students, and teaching. Older faculty members mentor younger ones, and sons follow fathers into the profession.

Steve Gluckman, John Pryor, I. S. Ravdin and Truman Schnabel are a few of the many punctuation points in a lineage of great medical teaching and mentoring at the University of Pennsylvania's medical school—a lineage that extends all the way back to its founding faculty at the dawn of America. Drs. John Morgan and Edward Shippen, about whom we'll talk more in the next section of the book, were both Surgeons General of Washington's revolutionary army.

Steve had one last piece of sound advice for the 163 newly frocked medical students at the Annenberg Center on Friday, the thirteenth of August, in 2010: "Make time for yourself and your family."

Mary Schmich says: "Get to know your parents. You never know when they'll be gone for good. Be nice to your siblings. They're your best link to your past and the people most likely to stick with you in the future." Steve's advice refers to how critical a healthy family life is to the maintenance of a sense of balance in a medical career. And his "Make time for yourself" is her "Dance, even if you have nowhere to do it but your living room."

The thing about Steve's address that struck me most as I listened to it weeks later was its timelessness. Every single thing he said, every lesson, would have applied equally well in 1810, 1910 or 2010. Hippocrates had a shorter version: "First, Do No Harm."

PART II

HISTORIES OF
MEDICINE

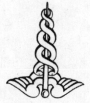

Medicine is among the oldest of professions. Holes in the skulls of pre-historic men, with healed bone, show evidence of the first successful neurosurgical procedures. We have no idea why these "trepanations" were performed—perhaps to let out evil spirits. Based on what we know now, the theories that guided medicine through much of its history were incorrect and often resulted in more harm than good. It's quite likely that the same will be said in the future of what we do now.

The profession has gone through periods in the past of substantial upheaval, much like the present. And the influence of individuals, some of whom were doctors and some of whom weren't, has shaped it in unexpected ways.

In this part of the book, we'll meet two ambitious young men who were once fast friends but became mortal enemies as they pursued their medical careers at the dawning of America. We'll see how the "goings about" of a former high school teacher at the beginning of the twentieth century changed medicine permanently and set it off toward the future we live in today. We'll meet the Hollywood doctors who served as role models for generations of future medical students. And we'll see how the lives of two sons of immigrants entwined during the upheavals of the Great Depression and World War II, resulting in a brand new model of medicine.

Finally, we'll see how the anguish of a father, and the light he shed on medical training, eventually led to the end of the medical apprenticeship and to a dramatic shift in the balance of power between the trainee and his teacher.

CHAPTER 6

DEAD PRESIDENTS

On the evening of Saturday, December 14, 1799, just days before the dawn of the nineteenth century, a previously active and healthy 67-year-old man lay dying in his bedroom. He was surrounded by no fewer than three doctors, his wife and his private secretary, who recorded for posterity many of the details of his illness and its treatments.

The two days before had been cold and snowy, and the man had been out and about in the weather, riding across the grounds of his estate. He returned on Thursday afternoon with his hair still covered in snow and proceeded directly to dinner, still wet. On Friday the thirteenth, he developed a sore throat but gamely went out again that afternoon to mark some trees he wished to be felled. That evening, he retired late to his bed after having reviewed some paperwork with his secretary. His wife evidently waited up for him until nearly midnight and chided him for staying up late when he was ill. According to the secretary, who presumably wasn't there, his response was: "I came so soon as my business was accomplished. You well know that through a long life, it has been my unvaried rule, never to put off till tomorrow the duties which should be performed today."[1] The increasingly ill man must have croaked out that fine speech, for he awakened his wife in the wee hours, barely able to speak and complaining of "ague," which was the term used at the time to describe the combination of fever, chills and shivering.

The man's sore throat may have been merely viral in origin, but some of the alternative diagnoses that have been proposed in subsequent analyses include quinsy, the term for what we now call a *peritonsillar abscess*;

cynanche trachealis—what we would call strep throat; and epiglottitis, a bacterial infection of the entrance to the trachea. Whatever the cause, the patient's pain and breathing worsened during the early hours of Saturday morning. When the chambermaid arrived to light the fire in the bedroom, the patient summoned the overseer of his farm, George Rawlins. Rawlins had some practical veterinary experience, and the man bade him take some blood from a vein—a common all-purpose remedy of the day. His wife looked on anxiously lest too much be drained and made sure his feet were bathed in warm water. She tied a flannel soaked in smelling salts around his neck.

These relatively mild ministrations were unsuccessful, and real doctors, who had been urgently summoned, eventually arrived on horseback from several points of the compass. The first, Dr. James Craik, took more blood and applied a cantharides plaster to the patient's throat over the most obviously diseased area.

Cantharides, considered a medication at that time, was derived from a chemical called *cantharidin*, which is produced by a beautiful, emerald-green beetle commonly known as the Spanish fly. A powder made from crushed Spanish-fly beetles is often given orally, even today, to farm animals as a sexual stimulant and has been used for centuries in various forms by humans for the same purpose. When consumed by an animal or a human, the cantharidin is eventually excreted in the urine, causing a burning irritation of the urinary tract and inflammation of the genitals.

The Marquis de Sade is said to have given prostitutes candies laced with Spanish fly at an orgy in 1772, and was consequently sentenced to death for poisoning and subsequent sodomy. The sentence was later reprieved by the king, although the Marquis did spend many years in prison for this and other crimes. Much of the salacious writing for which he is most well known was done in prison—where he was unable to engage in anything more than an active fantasy life.

When cantharides is applied to the skin, rather than taken internally, it causes blistering. This was the effect desired by Dr. Craik when he prescribed the plaster treatment for his patient. Craik presumably intended to draw "bad humors" from the inflammation on the inside of the throat through the overlying skin by raising a therapeutic blister on it. The cantharides plaster that Craik applied to his patient would have produced, in sequence, a tingling sensation, redness, pain and finally the development of a fluid-filled vesicle on the skin beneath the plaster. The fluid was then drained by the physician in a process called an *evacuation*.

As it happened, Dr. Craik's interventions were no more successful than those of the overseer Rawlins, and he called for additional help. By mid-afternoon, two more doctors, Elisha Dick and Jerome Brown, joined him in consultation. But Craik had not been idle in the meantime, having applied more cantharides plasters to the patient's legs and feet and brewed up a gargle of vinegar and sage tea. Unfortunately, this mouthwash nearly suffocated the man, and Craik's prescription for the inhalation of steam did little more than stimulate a coughing spell.

Drs. Dick and Brown felt the pulse and examined the throat of the increasingly ill man, and the doctors then retired as a group to discuss. That afternoon of the fourteenth had turned severely cold, so the three wise men were undoubtedly clustered around a fire and understandably extremely anxious as to the fate of their patient. Dr. Dick was the youngest of them and counseled against one proposed course of action as the patient worsened, saying, "He has already been bled three times today....He needs all of his strength and further bleeding will diminish it."[2] However, in the end, the two older doctors prevailed. More bloodletting was prescribed, but they noted that the blood "flowed less well from the vein" on this fourth attempt. This is not surprising to us today, because, as we know now, almost half of the patient's blood volume had been drained in merely a few hours.

Undaunted, the doctors pulled out all the stops. They prescribed both calomel and tartar, taking a belt-and-suspenders approach to the purging of the patient. Calomel is the chemical *mercurous chloride*, which was used routinely as a laxative by physicians of the era to release impurities from the body. What no one realized back then was that this treatment actually caused the teeth and hair of many patients to fall out. Tartar emetic, the other drug, is a white powder with a sweetish metallic taste that contains potassium and antimony. Tartar causes vomiting, salivation and sweating, and, as with calomel, it was thought at the time to eliminate impurities in the body.

By late evening of the fourteenth, the patient lay ashen and exhausted from illness, blood loss, blistering, vomiting and diarrhea. His sickroom would have reeked of the combined odors of smoke, vomit, bile and stool as well as the coppery smell of blood. There would have been little dignity left for the man, yet he apparently had strength enough to indicate that one of the two wills in his desk should be burnt and the other preserved. Near the end, he whispered, "Let my corpse be kept for the usual period of three days." And then, according to the witnesses: "Composing his form at length, and folding his arms on his bosom, without a sigh, without a groan, the Father of his Country died. No pang or struggle told when the noble spirit took its noiseless flight."[3] George Washington was the first dead president.

It's hard to imagine exactly what it must have been like in Washington's death room on that cold night. By our standards, his would have been a relatively sudden death. He had been out on the grounds of Mount Vernon on his horse the afternoon before and was dead 24 hours later despite everything a bevy of doctors could do. Today, we would almost certainly have cured him with a single dose of antibiotics, and we certainly wouldn't have bled, blistered or purged. But deaths of this sort were, sadly, not uncommon in the late 1700s; and patients were indeed able, on occasion, to orchestrate their death, as Washington did, even as they lay dying.

Medical historians believe that Washington was killed by the combined effects of blood-letting and the additional fluid losses from blisters, vomiting and diarrhea—all of which was compounded by his inability to take any liquids by mouth because of his inflamed throat. In fact, according to the modern Advanced Trauma Life Support system for the classification of blood loss, Washington's physicians drained enough blood to put him in Class III hypovolemic shock, the symptoms of which are very fast heart and respiratory rates, cool clammy skin, low blood pressure, anxiety and agitation. It is a testament to Washington's force of will that he was able under these circumstances to manage the events around him to a large degree.

Medicine was still a young discipline in America in 1799, and there were few doctors and even fewer hospitals. In fact, the oldest patient care facility in the not-yet-united states was created by some of Washington's fellow founding fathers. On May 11, 1751, a charter was granted by the Pennsylvania Assembly to establish the first hospital in the Americas, in Philadelphia.[4] The project was conceived of by Dr. Thomas Bond, a Quaker who moved to Philadelphia from Maryland as a young man. Like many medical men of his era, Bond's initial medical training took place in England and France. While in the latter, he became familiar with the new "hospital movement" exemplified by the *Hôtel-Dieu* in Paris. It was part of France's network of what were called *hostels of God*, established primarily as health-care facilities for the poor. The *Hôtel-Dieu* was originally founded by Saint Landry, the then-bishop of Paris, in 651 AD and still operates today, almost fifteen centuries later, as the *Hôpital Hôtel-Dieu* on the Ile de la Cité across the street from the cathedral of Notre Dame.

After his education abroad, Dr. Bond returned to practice in Philadelphia, which was to become the second-largest English-speaking city in the British Empire prior to the American Revolution. Philadelphia's Delaware River port was already a major shipping center, from which meat, flour and lumber were sent to Europe in return for manufactured goods and wine from the Old World. Americans, Europeans, American Indians and Africans mingled freely along the waterfront of the river. Not surprisingly, this cosmopolitan population exchanged diseases from all over the world just as freely as they mingled, and by a variety of transmission routes.

While Philadelphia was a prosperous town due to its commerce, the prosperity was not divided equally among its inhabitants. As with large cities from the dawn of humanity, there were poor, sick, injured and mentally ill who wandered its streets, often uncared for. Thomas Bond "conceived of the idea of establishing a hospital in Philadelphia for the reception and cure of poor sick persons," much like the Parisian *hôpital* at which he had trained.[5]

However, the concept of any kind of hospital was new to Philadelphians. In response to Bond's proposal, the city leadership asked him to determine what Benjamin Franklin, the city's intellectual leader, thought of the idea. Franklin turned out to be both enthusiastic and supportive—he eventually went on to write the cornerstone inscription for the east wing of the new hospital's Pine Building. That edifice still stands today, acting both as administrative space and a museum for the very active Pennsylvania Hospital. The inscription on the still-visible Franklin cornerstone reads in part: "This Building, By the bounty of the Government And of Many private Persons, Was piously founded, For the Relief of the Sick and Miserable."[6]

Franklin's 1751 petition to the state assembly in support of its establishment, entitled "Appeal for the Hospital," contains the statement: "The Good particular Men may do separately...is small compared with what they may do collectively." Reminiscing later about the hospital's origins, Franklin said, "I do not remember any of my political manoeuvres, the success of which gave me at the time more pleasure."[7] To be fair, while Franklin founded many things and is often given credit for this hospital, its establishment was primarily Bond's work. Dr. Bond went on to serve on its staff until his death. He has been described as "the father of clinical medicine" in America.[8]

In the seventeenth and early eighteenth centuries, the medical education of a young doctor, in both Europe and the New World, typically occurred during a period of apprenticeship to a reputable practitioner. The trainee started as a menial, running errands, feeding horses, cleaning bottles and wrangling leeches. With time, the scope of his responsibilities increased, and he came to mix the medicines and roll out the plasters—mustard and cantharides plasters (like those utilized on Washington) were used, for example, to draw circulation to the skin. At the end of his term of indenture, the trainee began to participate in actual patient care, doing small surgical procedures, perhaps pulling teeth, leeching or draining blood by scarification of the skin with a sharp instrument.

By the mid-eighteenth century, more ambitious physicians began to travel to medical schools in Scotland, France, England, Belgium and Sweden, as did Philadelphia's Thomas Bond. The graduates of these schools eventually went on to become the founders of new medical schools in the United States. Philadelphia was the center in America of both medicine and commerce in the mid-1700s. It was there that William Shippen Jr. became the city's first teacher of anatomy, surgery and obstetrics. He and his physician father, William Shippen Sr., would both eventually become medical staff members at Bond's new Pennsylvania Hospital.

After apprenticing with his father until 1758, the younger Shippen earned his medical degree at the University of Edinburgh and subsequently returned to Philadelphia in 1762. One of the first things he did upon his return was to announce a series of anatomical lectures "for the advantage of the young gentleman now engaged in the study of physic," in other words, for the medical apprentices of the day, "whose circumstances and connections will not admit of their going abroad for improvement to the anatomical schools of Europe; and also for the entertainment of any gentlemen who may have the curiosity to understand the human frame."[9] With this latter declaration, Shippen effectively offered to open his lessons and the bodies of human cadavers to the prurient eyes of the general public.

His demonstrations were advertised in the *Pennsylvania Gazette*, an early American newspaper published by Benjamin Franklin, as follows: "Dr. Shippen's anatomical lectures will begin tomorrow evening, at six o'clock, at his father's house in Fourth Street. Tickets for the course to be had of the doctor at five pistoles each; and any gentlemen who incline to see the subject prepared for the lectures, and learn the art of dissecting, injecting, etc., are to pay five pistoles more."[10]

A ticket to Shippen's course was stamped with a red wax seal and signed by the doctor himself. It read, "Admit the bearer [to] Doctor Shippen's Anatomical Lectures," which included anatomical drawings and casts by Jan Van Rymsdyk, the famous Dutch painter. Shippen also offered a second course on midwifery to both women and men, which was almost certainly an equally sensational draw. His ostensible motive was the elevation of midwifery from a job performed by "unskilled old women" and involving "the dangerous and cruel use of instruments," to a true medical discipline performed by physicians. However, some of the conservative Quaker population of Philadelphia found the concept of a male midwife offensive, so Shippen's lectures were periodically interrupted by mobs or stones thrown through the windows.[11]

Accused at one point of grave robbing from a local church burial ground, Shippen defended himself saying that he had only dissected the bodies of "suicides, executed felons, and now and then the one from the Potter's Field."[12] In fact, the Shippen residence became so notorious that it was made the subject of a song sung by schoolboys, who feared the place as the home of ghosts and evil doctors and chanted:

> The body-snatchers! They have come
>   And made a snatch at me;
> It's very hard them kind of men
>   Won't let a body be!
> Don't go to weep upon my grave,
>   And think that there I'll be;
> They haven't left an atom there
>   Of my anatomy.[13]

The turmoil and ferment attending these beginnings of medicine in the New World extended beyond Shippen's classroom. While Shippen would eventually be appointed the first professor of anatomy and surgery in the newly formed College of Philadelphia's Medical School, the school's actual founder was his one-time good friend and fellow Edinburgh graduate, John Morgan, who was appointed professor of the theory and practice of medicine at the college in May 1765, several months before Shippen's election to the faculty. Here again, Ben Franklin played a major organizational role. As one of the college's original founders in 1749, Franklin was well positioned to support the establishment of a medical faculty within it and to determine the faculty's composition.

The College of Philadelphia is now known as the University of Pennsylvania, and its medical school was the first in the colonies. John Morgan and William Shippen the Younger were both determined young men. Although they started as friends, they ultimately became lifelong enemies following their competition over the establishment of the medical school, eventually feuding over a variety of issues. Their quarrel started when Shippen claimed that Morgan stole his idea for a new medical school in the soon-to-be capital of the New World. Morgan and Shippen were born within a year of one another, and both went to the Nottingham Academy, a private undergraduate school located outside of Philadelphia in Chester County. Shippen went on to graduate as valedictorian from Princeton College, while Morgan was educated at the College of Philadelphia before it had a medical faculty. Both eventually found themselves at Edinburgh's medical school, which had origins extending back to the early 1500s with the incorporation of the Barber Surgeons of Edinburgh, a craft guild. Both of these very ambitious young men eventually returned to Philadelphia, where they would compete continuously until one of them finally died.[14]

Morgan was, perhaps, the more farsighted of the two. Rather than returning directly from Edinburgh to Philadelphia after his studies in Scotland, he traveled to Paris for additional polishing. He visited the pope in Rome with the Duke of York in the spring of 1764 and subsequently became a fellow of the Royal Academy of Surgery in Paris, the Royal College of Physicians of Edinburgh, as well as London's Royal College of Physicians, before returning to Pennsylvania. Armed with these impressive Old World credentials, Morgan immediately eclipsed the already locally established Shippen despite the fact that the latter was a fourth-generation Philadelphian. Morgan was able to persuade the trustees of the College of Philadelphia to establish a medical faculty shortly after his triumphant return. And while Shippen and Morgan had agreed to work together toward that end while still students in Scotland, it was Morgan who took the initiative and received the credit. Although he invited Shippen to become the second member of the new faculty several months later, his old friend was miffed.

Morgan went on to become a founding member of the American Philosophical Society, a scholarly group conceived of by Benjamin Franklin that is still in existence in Philadelphia today and now includes over 200 Nobel prize winners among its past and present membership. In what must have been perceived as yet one more slight to Shippen, Morgan was named Director-General of the Revolutionary army's Boston-based hospital—an act of the newly formed Congress in 1775, at the outset of the American Revolution. In this new role, the still-young physician was immediately confronted with an outbreak of smallpox, a shortage of supplies and a general lack of understanding about sanitation and disease on the part of both the army and the Congress. These problems were, not surprisingly, attributed to failures on the part of the new Director-General. Sensing weakness, Shippen was quick to undermine Morgan, eventually proposing his own plan for reorganizing the army medical department. In April 1777, Congress abruptly relieved Morgan of his title and replaced him with Shippen.

Within six months of Shippen's coup, a third prominent Philadelphia physician, Dr. Benjamin Rush, described the newest Director-General as being both "ignorant and negligent in his duty."[15] He and Morgan accused Shippen of malpractice and misconduct in his office—claims that were brought before Congress and the army high command. Shippen was eventually arrested on charges that he had speculated with precious supplies such as sugar and wine that were originally intended for sick and wounded soldiers. During the trial, it became clear that despite being the physician-in-chief, Shippen never visited the sick, provided comfort nor dressed the soldiers' wounds. He was eventually acquitted of the charges by a military review board, but there were clear irregularities in its conduct; Shippen, for example, entertained the board with fine food and mocked Morgan to them. However, having lost credibility as a result of his conduct, Shippen resigned his post shortly after the trial.

Morgan attempted to repair his own damaged reputation in a tract entitled "Vindication of His Public Character," and his efforts were ultimately rewarded with a statement from a congressional subcommittee, which concluded that Morgan "did conduct himself ably and faithfully in the discharge of the duties of his office, [and] therefore Resolved that Congress are satisfied with the conduct of Doctor John Morgan while acting as the Director-General and Physician-in-Chief in the general hospitals of the United States."[16] Nevertheless, despite this testimonial, and exhausted, perhaps by his long feud with his one-time friend, Morgan never fully recovered his youthful vitality. He died in 1789 at the age of 53. Shippen, however, lived on well beyond his old foe and died at the ripe old age of 72 in 1808.

Despite the inauspicious, often-contentious beginnings of medicine in the New World, Shippen, Morgan and Rush, among others, worked together in 1787 to form the College of Physicians of Philadelphia, which was modeled after Europe's various Royal Colleges. In fact, Shippen's medicine chest can still be seen today in the college's Mutter Museum, which has a collection of over twenty thousand medical artifacts. The mission of the college is to uphold "the ideals and heritage of medicine," and the medical oddities on display in the museum include a plaster cast of the once world-famous Siamese twins, Chang and Eng, as well as the tallest skeleton in North America.

The medical chests of several of the college founders, including those of Shippen, his father and Benjamin Rush, are all part of the Mutter collection and represent a window on the medical technologies available at the time of the American Revolution. The chests' contents include apothecary scales, syringes, glass bottles, beakers and the traditional mortar and pestle. There are also cupping cups, which were heated and applied to the skin of a patient, drawing blood to the surface as they cooled and the air within them contracted. In fact, cupping is a traditional medical treatment that is still practiced in some areas of the world today and intended, at least theoretically, to address certain kinds of diseases thought to be due to cold and damp conditions.

Colonial physicians also used an assortment of drugs. The medical chests displayed at the Mutter Museum carried whiskey, brandy and wine, as well as ether. Interestingly, while ether was used medicinally in the Revolutionary War era, it was not yet recognized as an anesthetic agent; its use in that role had to wait until 1842. Paregoric, however, was in widespread use in the 1700s, as was its cousin laudanum. These opium-derived drugs come from the same family as morphine and heroin. The active narcotic ingredient is extracted from the latex produced within the seedpod of the poppy plant, which grew freely around Philadelphia at the time.

Paregoric was used to treat diarrhea and cough and to calm "fretful" children—maybe those who would today be described as having an attention deficit disorder, while laudanum was more often used as an analgesic, and like all narcotics, frequently became a drug of abuse. Cinnamon, caraway and lavender were probably included in the medicinal chests of the founding physicians for their favorable odors. There was a variety of metal-containing medications, such as iron filings, mercurial ointment and the calomel and tartar used as purgatives in the care of George Washington.

Physicians of the era based their diagnoses on theories extending back to the Greco-Roman physician Galen, who lived between 129 and 200 CE. Galen believed that imbalances in the body's "humors" (the basic substances he believed the human body was composed of) caused disease. According to Galenic medicine, a syndrome attributed to an excess of blood would be treated with blood-letting of some sort, while a disease attributed to excesses of cold and wet would be handled by interventions like cupping that brought blood to the surface. So, for example, if one had a fever and looked flushed, leeching or some other method of bleeding would have been prescribed to drain out some of the blood, while if one had a "cold," or looked pale and clammy, cupping or the application of a plaster was the very thing to bring the blood to the surface and improve the complexion.

Nearly 100 years after George Washington's death, Abraham Lincoln was shot in the head while enjoying a theatrical performance—a catastrophic injury that his physicians treated, at least in part, by inserting long metal probes into the skull defect. With each probing, blood and brain apparently oozed out. Between the doctors' interventions and the original wound, Lincoln, like Washington, lost a good deal of blood in the waning hours of his life. Despite the passage of a century between their terms as president, medicine had advanced little, and Lincoln's ashen coloring after the assassination prompted his doctors to prescribe the application of hot water bottles and blistering plasters to improve the circulation, just as Washington's doctors had done.

Lincoln would almost certainly have died even today from the gunshot or suffered permanent, incapacitating neurologic deficits. Washington, however, was killed by his caregivers—or, at the very least, hastened to his death. But it is worth noting that the treatments both received had their roots in medical theories first proposed by Galen shortly after the death of Christ.

The pharmacopeia (drugs) prescribed by physicians of the eighteenth, nineteenth and even early twentieth centuries were designed to remedy humoral imbalances. These interventions were based upon Galen's *theory* about the causes of disease rather than from empiric, scientific observation of the relationship between systematic applications of a treatment and its results. While most physicians over those centuries had unquestioning faith in Galen's theories and remedies, a few, such as the poet and physician Dr. Oliver Wendell Holmes (who was also the father of an American Supreme Court justice) ultimately became skeptical. In fact, Holmes once said waggishly that the entire *materia medica,* the medicinal drugs of his era, should be thrown into the sea (with the notable exceptions of opium, wine and ether), where it would be "all the better for mankind, and all the worse for the fishes."[17] Holmes also wrote:

> Science is a first-rate piece of furniture for a man's upper chamber,
> if he has common sense on the ground floor.

And,

> Many people die with their music still in them. Why is this so? Too
> often it is because they are always getting ready to live. Before they
> know it, time runs out.[18]

By the end of the nineteenth century, it had finally become apparent to astute observers of medicine (like Holmes) that Galen's theories and the treatments based upon them were seriously flawed and unscientific, particularly when compared to the major scientific breakthroughs that were being made contemporaneously in the worlds of chemistry, physics and biology. There was a growing sentiment among thoughtful doctors, and their patients, that it was time for the establishment of scientifically based approaches to the study, diagnosis and treatment of disease.

In 1910, the eponymously named foundation endowed by Andrew Carnegie five years earlier issued the first of a series of papers on professional schools in the United States, Canada and Newfoundland. Medical schools were the subject of the foundation's first publication, and the paper subsequently came to be known as the Flexner Report.[19] It revolutionized the education of medical students and as a consequence medical care in the decades following its release. In that period, largely as a result of the report and new regulations resulting from its recommendations, half of the nation's 160 medical schools closed, including three of the five schools dedicated to the education of black physicians.

The report also advocated the closure of the only three women's medical schools in existence at the time. The Flexner Report ultimately precipitated the transition from an era when most medical education occurred at proprietary schools, operated primarily for profit, to today's model where medical schools combine rigorous biomedical sciences with hands-on clinical training.

Abraham Flexner had been a high school principal for 20 years before he had a mid-career epiphany and subsequently went to graduate school at Harvard and the University of Berlin. He was then hired by the newly formed Carnegie Foundation. At the time he joined the foundation, he was an unemployed former schoolmaster who had run out of money and had no medical qualifications. In fact, he had never visited a medical school prior to starting his inquiry, but Flexner knew how to research a topic. During the course of his 18-month-long investigation, he visited 155 medical schools, sometimes seeing more than one per day.

He was hard driving and criticized by some contemporaries as "erratic, hard to get along with and somewhat uncertain in judgment." In fact, the then-president of Harvard University, Charles Eliot, said that "in controversial matters [Flexner] arouses strong opposition, partly...by his aspect of eagerness and partly by a certain satirical humor," and that "negotiation in matters which divide opinion strongly is not Mr. Flexner's forte."[20]

While Abraham Flexner was a staunch proponent of the scientific method, he had no rigorous or standard method of his own for evaluating the schools he visited. He relied heavily on casual observation. As he said, the "inconsistency never bothered me."[21] In fact, Flexner's personal motto was *ambulando discimus,* which is Latin for "We learn by going about." The record doesn't speak to whether or not he intended that "we" be taken in the royal sense, but, capricious and arrogant as Flexner may have been personally, his report revolutionized medicine.

The Flexner Report was issued a century ago, during a period when commercialism had, in the view of the study's author and the sponsoring foundation, so tainted medical education that doctors were not highly regarded. The variety of squabbling schools of medical education and practice included allopathy (what we would call *today's form of medicine*), in which remedies produce effects different from or opposite to those of the treated disease), homeopathy (in which remedies produce effects *similar* to the disease at issue), osteopaths (who used manipulation in their repertoire), eclectics (who used botanical remedies) and physiomedicals (who used physical rather than medicinal interventions).

There was also an abundance of doctors. Flexner describes the "overproduction of ill trained men...due to the existence of a very large number of commercial schools, sustained in many cases by advertising methods through which a mass of unprepared youth is drawn out of industrial occupations into the study of medicine," and the "clerk who is receiving $50 a month in the country store...gets an alluring brochure which paints the life of a physician as an easy road to wealth."

Flexner believed that the excess of practitioners "was worse than waste, for the superfluous doctor is usually a poor doctor." Distinct from Germany at the time, where there was "one doctor for every 2000 souls, and in the large cities one for every 1000," the United States had "on the average one doctor for every 568 persons" in 1909, and "many small towns with less than 200 inhabitants each [had] two or three physicians apiece."[22]

Similar discrepancies exist today in the patient-to-doctor ratio around the world ranging from 400-to-1 in much of the Western world to an appalling 50,000-to-1 ratio in parts of sub-Saharan Africa.[23] In the United States, proportions vary from approximately 200-to-1 along the Eastern Seaboard to 600-to-1 in parts of the Far West like Idaho and Nevada.[24] Interestingly, there is no evidence that having access to a higher density of today's doctors equates to better health care; and, indeed, there is an abundance of data showing that a higher doctor-patient ratio correlates with higher health-care costs. In fact, there are substantial differences between health-care expenditures in high-consumption locales like Miami, Manhattan and Los Angeles when compared to cities where medical costs tend to be lower, like Minneapolis, San Francisco and Rochester, New York, with no appreciable difference in medical outcomes for the patients.[25]

We are currently entering an epoch that will be as transformative to medicine as were the eras of Flexner and the feuding Shippen and Morgan, one and two centuries ago. Health-care costs are spiraling out of control on the one hand, while a host of new technologies hold unimaginable promise on the other. With the advent of electronic health records, telehealth, smart medical machines, genomics, personalized medicine, stem-cell therapies and nanotechnology, the practice of medicine is changing irreversibly. And so are the jobs of its practitioners. In the rest of this book, we'll explore the ways in which the practice of medicine will change as these new technologies mature.

Oliver Wendell Holmes made this eloquent statement:

One's mind, once stretched by a new idea, never regains its original dimensions.[26]

This quotation aptly describes both the promises and the dilemmas of medicine today. With each new medical discovery, we open Pandora's box a bit further. Our minds have become "stretched" to believe that, through relentless medical advances, we can defeat disease and mortality. A prevalent expectation is that medicine can mop up after our collective bad behaviors, such as eating poorly, smoking, drinking and drugging.

To date, at least, the sky has been the limit on what we've been willing to spend for health care, as evidenced by the relentless increases in medical expenditures as a percentage of the overall economies of modern societies. It has finally become clear, however, that we will need to shrink our stretched expectations, or—preferably—find new delivery models that will permit us to deliver on the seemingly limitless promise of medical progress in an affordable fashion.

CHAPTER 7

GO FORTH AND MULTIPLY

Like many couples, my wife Beth and I took our first tentative step into the world of creature rearing with the acquisition of a pet. I don't think we really thought about it in those terms at the time, but we adopted a male English Springer Spaniel puppy not too long after we married. We named him Chaos.

Even in retrospect, nothing about having done this seems terribly misguided. He was a good dog—not really chaotic at all. However, the next addition to the household clearly came about when we were in the grip of some kind of mutual madness. We had learned several months earlier that we were soon to be parents of human twins. And yet, for reasons that are completely opaque today, we decided to take in a second Springer Spaniel puppy a couple of months before the twins were expected to join us. We called *this* dog Mayhem—aptly, as it turned out, because in short order we went from a mostly sedate household to a house full of creatures with a range of special needs.

Springers were the founding breed of the English hunting spaniels. They have a great sense of smell and were specifically bred to track and then flush game birds like pheasants and woodcocks into the air from hunkered-down positions in the brush. Spaniels appear in paintings dating all the way back to the 1500s, when birds of prey like falcons were used to kill and retrieve the flushed bird for the hunter, and hunting was done for food rather than for sport.

In fact, spaniels may have come to the British Isles as early as the time of Christ. They are believed to have originated from what was then called Hispania but is now known as the Iberian Peninsula. After the development of the shotgun, spaniels continued to serve as hunting companions, enabling the landed gentry to shoot flushed game birds on the wing.

Today, the range of hunting spaniels includes the Cocker, Russian, English, French, German, Irish and Welsh variants and, more recently, the Sprocker (a Springer/Cocker crossbreed). They're all descendants of the progenitor generic spaniel, and many of these nationally specific varieties have further split into distinct *field* and *show* sub-breeds, where the latter are what can only be described as prettier. The field Springer, for example, is smaller and has a short, coarse coat, while the show version has luxurious, often wavy, liver or black hair. The short, coarse coat of the field dog protects the dog from the often thorny, burry underbrush through which it hunts; the longer hair of the show breed turns into a tangled mess in those same conditions but shows well under the lights at a dog show like the Westminster Kennel Club's annual canine beauty pageant. And while field and show Springers are still registered as a single breed, the two varieties have in reality become so differentiated that the gene pools are quite distinct. Functionally speaking, a field Springer would not fare well in a dog show, and a show dog would not have the stamina, nose or speed to do well in a field trial.

Today's doctors are just as differentiated as dogs. The same selective species diversification and specialization has occurred explosively in medicine in the decades since Flexner's report at the beginning of the twentieth century. Like dogs, physicians can trace their origins back to one common ancestor—Hippocrates is generally regarded as the *ur*-Physician in Western medicine. And much as a show Springer bears very little resemblance to that first domesticated wolf from which all dogs sprang, today's physician specialists are a far cry from the Hippocratic model, despite the fact that we have all recited some version of the Hippocratic oath at some point in our careers.

The medical profession has differentiated into a range of highly specialized breeds such as the interventional neuroradiologist, the transplant hepatologist and, more recently, the bariatric surgeon. The original practitioners in each of these fields were merely *sub*-specialists—just bariatric surgeon, transplant or abdominal surgeons. They, in turn, derived their respective ancestries from even less specialized radiologists, gastroenterologists and general surgeons. But with the passage of time and a kind of selective breeding, these more highly evolved forms have emerged.

We're even beginning to see medical *cross*breeds—analogous to the canine Sprocker. For example, a neuro*surgeon* may integrate the skills of an interventional neuro*radiologist* into his practice, and cardiac *surgeons* employ techniques designed by cardiologists in some of the newest valve-replacement procedures. The names for these new specialties have not yet been created, but when they are, they'll certainly be tongue-twisters.

Just as paintings chronicled the origins of specific canine species, the life-and-death stories of patients and the doctors and nurses who care for them have been endlessly captured in more-modern media, such as books, movies and television, since the early years of the twentieth century, giving us a living record of the evolution of today's physician. There has always been a complicated interplay between the fictional medical characters depicted by screenwriters, the impact their shows have had on public perceptions of the profession and the medical profession's reaction to these medical dramas.

The *Dr. Kildare* movies of the 1930s; *The Donna Reed Show* and *Hennesey* in the 1950s; *Ben Casey, Dr. Kildare, The Fugitive* and *Marcus Welby, M.D.* in the 1960s; *Bold Ones, Medical Center, Emergency, M.D., M*A*S*H* and *Quincy, M.E.* in the 1970s; *The Cosby Show, St. Elsewhere, Doogie Howser, M.D.* and *Trapper John, M.D.* in the 1980s; *E.R.* and *Chicago Hope* in the 1990s and, most recently, shows like *Grey's Anatomy, House* and *Nip/Tuck*—all have simultaneously portrayed and subtly shaped medicine over the course of the past century. And whereas the early series strove for an American Medical Association stamp of approval, more recent dramas have clearly veered toward the fantastical—departing at times almost gleefully from any semblance of medical reality. Of course, true medical reality shows have proliferated to fill that void.

The first Dr. Kildare movie was entitled *Internes Can't Take Money* and was based on a story sold to *Cosmopolitan* magazine by one of America's most prolific pulp writers, Frederick Schiller Faust, who used the pen name Max Brand. The story features a young, poor country-boy-turned-medical-trainee named Jimmie Kildare. Kildare is a Depression-era hero, a hardworking, honorable young professional who, when offered money for saving the life of a gangster, replies that "interns can't take money." The movie costars a popular actor named Joel McCrea with Barbara Stanwyck as the love interest (she went on to win an honorary Academy

Award for her roles in television and movies, including *The Big Valley* and *The Thorn Birds*).

The first Kildare movie was both successful at the box office and well-reviewed, and Paramount Pictures eventually went on to make a series of ten Kildare films, including *Young Dr. Kildare, Calling Dr. Kildare* and *Dr. Kildare's Strange Case.* In these films, Kildare is equally comfortable in the roles of surgeon, orthopedist, internist, family practitioner and psychiatrist. In each, he is paired up with an older doctor named Leonard Gillespie, who counterbalances Kildare's youth, inexperience and starry-eyed optimism with age, knowledge and curmudgeonliness. Lionel Barrymore played this role in most of the movies, and Raymond Massey took on a more fatherly version of the same character in the Dr. Kildare television series of the 1960s. The American Medical Association endorsed the Kildare movies' depiction of the heroic, multitalented young doctor, which was consistent with its desire to counter other less favorable movies of the era showing doctors as "avaricious" and "vultures."[1]

The original Dr. Kildare was a kind of medical Everyman, an undifferentiated Doctor, who was equally at home sewing up a life-threatening gash on a barroom table and diagnosing a case of hysterical blindness in a young heiress. Kildare's diverse range of competencies didn't raise an eyebrow in the 1930s and 1940s, but by the 1960s the concept of medical specialization had firmly taken root in the minds of screenwriters who created material for a new wave of medical television serials and often spent time in academic medical centers to prepare their scripts.

Dr. Kildare, as played by Richard Chamberlain on television, was a boyish, appealing ingénue, skilled in the art of human interaction. Chamberlain was *the* TV heartthrob of the 1960s and later went on to some success in big-screen movies such as *The Three Musketeers* and *The Count of Monte Cristo,* as well as in television miniserials like *The Thorn Birds.* From the American medical establishment's standpoint, Kildare was the perfect model doctor: handsome, hardworking and earnest, a resident in training to become a specialist in internal medicine.

Chamberlain became the male equivalent of a pinup model during the 1961–1966 run of the *Dr. Kildare* show. He described the double life he led during those years in his 2003 autobiography entitled *Shattered Love,* in which he admits that he hid his homosexuality in order to pursue his career as an actor. In contrast, the protagonist of *Ben Casey,* another popular medical television drama, was equally gruff and macho on and off the set. Vince Edwards arrived for his audition in a dirty tee shirt and with a several days' growth of beard. He was by all accounts difficult to manage on the set and best at playing angry.

Certain formulas were used over and over in these medical television series, and they, in turn, shaped public perception of what physicians did, how they acted and the environment in which they worked. One such theme was the relationship between the protagonist and an older physician mentor, like Dr. Gillespie in the Kildare dramas. Another was the invariably adversarial relationship between the physician and the medical administrator, with the latter usually trying to withhold scarce or costly resources from the former, and the former prevailing week after week. Comic relief might be embodied by a character such as the ambulance driver in the first Kildare movie, although the genre eventually spawned medically oriented comedy series, like *M*A*S*H*.

These programs also had a profound and fundamental impact on the profession itself by influencing the way in which real young doctors behaved, the perceptions of the young people who chose to go into the field and the often-unrealistic expectations patients came to have of their own physicians. For example, both Drs. Kildare and Welby were extraordinarily available and accommodating. According to Joseph Turow, the author of *Playing Doctor*,

The credo of [*Marcus Welby, M.D.*] was totally unrealistic for the modern physician. Focusing on one patient and his [or her] family per episode, Welby and [his sidekick] Kiley seemed to be running a two-person intensive care service. Their attendance to medical problems included spending much time counseling [the patient] and their family, driving them to the hospital, adjusting their oxygen, sitting with them through the night, and standing by in the operating room while the surgeon did his thing. Beyond these duties, the doctors found time to take patients to ball games, serve them elaborate dinners, stop by their workplaces, and attend their weddings.

And,

What stood for "hospital" in those series was the high-technology specialist orientation of the modern teaching institution [which]

pulsated with an awareness of, and a pride in, the inexorableness of medical progress. Acute life and death problems pumped dramatic adrenaline into a "damn the costs," immediate response atmosphere where physicians were kings.[2]

Ben Casey was a neurosurgeon in the show of that name, and his on-again, off-again love interest was an anesthesiologist. Marcus Welby was a family practitioner; Quincy, a pathologist; and Trapper John, a thoracic surgeon. Cliff Huxtable was an obstetrician on *The Cosby Show,* and Jason Seaver was a psychiatrist on *Growing Pains.* By the 1970s, the era of the medical specialist had arrived, and the distinct personalities of the specialists were used to drive the drama of the shows. Some doctors were nice "people-persons," others were gruff, some were funny, and others were acerbic—but they were all passionate about their work as evidenced by their ability to move mountains to save lives or, in the case of the forensic pathologist, to solve the seemingly impenetrable medical mysteries surrounding a death. The celebration of specialty medicine was at once a sign of the times and a spur to further medical differentiation.

The first medical specialty board was the American Board for Ophthalmic Examinations, which was incorporated in 1918, eight years after the issuance of the Flexner Report. The organization's name was later changed to the American Board of Ophthalmology. The American Board of Otorhinolaryngology, or what is sometimes called Ear, Nose and Throat medicine, was founded in 1924. The American Board of Obstetrics and Gynecology arose in 1930, and the American Board of Dermatology and Syphilology became the fourth such board in 1932.

By 1976, there were 22 specialty boards with 65 sub-specialties, according to a *New England Journal of Medicine* "Sounding Board" editorial entitled "Proliferation of Certification in Medical Specialties: Productive or Counterproductive?" In it, the author describes a "disturbing" cycle in which:

1) As a result of advances in a field or development of a new technology, a new group develops special expertise in this area.
2) An organization or society is formed for an exchange of ideas and to display advances to one another.

3) Membership in the organization becomes a mark of distinction in the field, and, in an effort to externalize that recognition, certification of excellence in the field becomes established.

4) Institutions with responsibility for quality of health care soon accept certification as evidence of competence and limit care within that field to those certified.[3]

The author, who was an official of the National Board of Examiners at the time, goes on to point out how referrals of complex patients to specialists by generalists is typically welcomed at the birth of a new specialty, but that, as time passes, an expectation develops that *any* patient with a problem in that specialty area, whether complex or routine, should be referred to the specialist. The generalist then begins to see fewer of what used to be routine patients, his comfort and perhaps competence in that area dwindle and the cycle becomes self-perpetuating. For example, whereas a general surgeon once handled a broad range of operations, many of those same operations are now performed by surgical specialists, like surgical oncologists—cancer surgeons—or hepatic surgeons who specialize in operations on the liver. Today more than 145 specialty or sub-specialty fields are recognized by the American Board of Medical Specialties.[4]

Orchid breeders, like dog breeders, are highly skilled at propagating new hybrid species with desirable characteristics like prettier flowers or resistance to pests. Orchidologists must work with a fastidious organism in warm, humid conditions and with seeds that contain no stored nourishment (unlike a typical fruit, for example). Much of the orchid breeder's work is done in a hothouse supplemented by plenty of fertilizer and water, where the conditions are ideal for the generation of new species from old ones. The greenhouses of medicine are academic medical centers and specialty hospitals, which have perfect conditions for the development of new subspecialist physicians from less well-differentiated parent species.

The conditions that led to the formation of the American Board of Ophthalmic Examinations early in the twentieth century perfectly illustrate the way in which new specialties develop to this day. At the turn of the century, ophthalmology was but one portion of a general practice in eye, ear, nose and throat medicine. The specialty hospitals of the era were, for example, the New York Eye and Ear Infirmary and the Illinois Eye and Ear Infirmary. It was with the development in 1913 of a handheld, battery-powered ophthalmoscope, which permitted relatively easy examination of the retina in the back of the eye, that the field blossomed.

While the previous version of the ophthalmoscope was a large, fixed machine, portable instruments could be used by family practitioners and other generalists. As they became more familiar with the use of the instrument, these generalists naturally discovered things in the back of the eye that they either couldn't explain or that were obviously abnormal. Some of the former were normal variants, and some of the latter were disease processes that perhaps hadn't yet affected the patient's vision enough for him to notice. Referrals by ophthalmoscope-wielding generalists to eye experts increased, and interest in the retina blossomed. New areas of research developed.

Eventually there was enough new opthalmologically based eye information to be mastered that eye practice diverged from ear, nose and throat practice, and the field of ophthalmology emerged as a distinct specialty.[5] And at a later time, the *sub*-specialty of neuro-ophthalmology further evolved from that root discipline of ophthalmology. Neuro-ophthalmology is the sub-specialty that deals with visual impairments due to brain pathology, such as the blindness caused by tumors in the brain's visual centers. This hybrid sub-specialty developed and matured in parallel with the field of neurosurgery, which had, in turn, diverged as a sub-specialty from general surgery.

Darwin's theory of evolution relies on the concept of continuous competition for resources. More-modern evolutionary biologists contend that cooperation and interaction among species are equally powerful forces. As one group put it, "Life did not take over the world by combat, but by networking."[6] The interaction between the neuro-ophthalmologist and the neurosurgeon is a good example of cooperative, non-Darwinian co-evolution of two medical species.

A neuro-ophthalmologist might evaluate a patient with blindness that is unexplained by direct examination of the eyes (because the eyes were normal) and might thereby identify the presence of a brain lesion requiring the services of a neurosurgeon. Similarly, the neurosurgeon might see a patient with a brain lesion based in the vision center and request the assistance of the neuro-opthalmologist in determining its effects on vision. The doctors in these two disciplines thereby developed what ecologists would call a *symbiotic relationship*—more specifically, a mutualistic symbiotic relationship wherein both parties benefited. They shared a "resource"—their patients—on which both depended.

In this example, the catalyst for the emergence of ophthalmology as a new specialty was that new technological device, the portable ophthalmoscope, which accelerated the discovery of new diagnoses and treatments in eye pathology. This same pattern has recurred repeatedly with other specialties. The periodic introduction of paradigm-changing technologies like the ophthalmoscope, ultrasound, CT scanning or magnetic resonance imaging has had the same effect on medical ecology that irrigation might have had on a previously arid patch of desert. The flora and fauna change rapidly and quickly following the introduction of the new technology. In cardiology, for example (a sub-specialty of internal medicine), advances in intravascular catheter technology led to the emergence of the *sub-sub*-specialty called *interventional cardiology*. Similarly, the development of ultrasound as a non-invasive technology allowing a doctor to "see" tissues inside the body preceded and permitted the development of cardiac ultrasonography, another sub-sub-specialty of cardiology. Electrophysiology, the sub-sub-specialty of cardiology that deals with heart rhythm problems, resulted from advances in pacemaker technology.

But this medical speciation is almost inevitably accompanied by extinction, just as in nature: some specialties, such as syphilology, have completely disappeared as effective treatments have eliminated the disease. Gone too are seizurists, retardationists and phrenologists.[7]

In the century since the Flexner Report was issued, we've seen dramatic increases in the amount of medical information. During this era, money has been plentiful and lots of talented young people have been attracted to the field, providing ideal growth conditions for medicine. It has made sense for medical schools to act as academic hothouses and to breed new hybrid medical fields. As a result, there has been an explosion of medical diversity: over 50 new sub-specialties were approved by the American Board of Medical Specialties between 1990 and 2009 alone. In retrospect, the advances in medicine during the twentieth century can be seen as analogous to the Cambrian explosion, an evolutionary period during which many complicated new animal groups appeared when previously there had been only relatively simple, single- or multi-celled organisms.

While the environment has seemingly been ideally suited for species diversification in medicine over much of the past century, we are now entering a new era in which previously lush financial resources will be sharply curtailed. This would suggest that progress will be slowed as a result.

However, technological advances in genomics, materials sciences, nano-technology and computer technology are poised to accelerate change. So it's hard to predict yet whether medical evolution is about to slow abruptly or perhaps change course dramatically, shucking off antiquated practices in the process, like an old skin. It may well be that there will be an entirely new set of medical evolutionary winners. Here again, we can look to nature's lessons for some insight.

The relationship between resource availability and species diversity in natural communities has been extensively studied by evolutionary biologists using a model known as *island biogeography*, which was developed by ecologists Robert MacArthur and E. O. Wilson in the 1960s. Wilson is the Pulitzer Prize–winning scientist and science essayist who has written extensively about, among many topics, the lessons that ant colonies have for humans.

Island biogeography explores factors contributing to species richness in an environment where resources are circumscribed by water or some other barrier. Ecologists use the terms *immigration* and *extinction* and propose that island biodiversity reaches equilibrium when these two forces are balanced. As one author put it, "Over the short term, competition for resources generates an equilibrium level of species diversity through a balance between immigration and extirpation. Over the longer term, equilibrium diversity reflects a balance between speciation and extinction, but in all cases the available resources control the equilibrium diversity."[8]

Although it is admittedly a bit of a stretch to compare natural environments like an island to the medical environment, there are instructive parallels. Some illnesses are, of course, caused by natural species, and over time diseases such as smallpox, syphilis, tuberculosis and malaria have become threatened or extinct in the medical ecosystem of modern society. As these diseases faded in significance, so did the specialists who would treat or research them. In other words, as syphilis disappeared as a public-health problem, there was no longer a need for syphilologists, resulting in a parallel extinction as their "food source" dried up. At the same time, new diseases—such as HIV, obesity and certain cancers—have "emigrated" from other species or arisen spontaneously in the same ecosystem—the medical island—and new specialists and specialties developed as a result. The epidemic of obesity, for example, begat the new field known as *bariatrics* and will be a robust new source of "resources" for medical providers in coming eras.

More recent work suggests that the degree of diversity in an ecosystem may not depend solely on the available resources, but that the degree of existing diversification may *itself* play an integral role in determining the degree of speciation on an island. In other words, the reason the tropics have so many species is that they have so many species. One explanation for this nonintuitive idea is that greater community complexity may drive greater diversity. Said another way: as species evolve, they create new ecological niches and expand the available eco-space. The greater complexity of the medical community in academic centers rich with specialists has driven medical diversification in the last century.

My Springer Spaniels—Chaos and Mayhem—both died at around the age of 12 years of diseases to which Springers are particularly susceptible. The seeds of their demise were carried in their genome, as is the case with many of today's dog species. The now relatively inbred Springer Spaniel has become particularly vulnerable to certain tumors and metabolic diseases. Many medical specialties suffer from this same kind of vulnerability.

A specialty's disease may go away, as with the syphilologist. Or some other specialty may "steal their bacon." Cardiac surgeons, for example, were once busily employed bypassing coronary arteries, but the cardiac surgical field is now stagnant. Strikingly, the average age of cardiac surgeons has increased from 50 to 57 as young people have stopped entering this once highly sought-after field.[9]

Unlike syphilis, coronary artery blockages haven't gone away; instead, cardiologists have developed techniques like balloon angioplasty and stenting, eliminating the need for surgery in many cases and leaving the cardiac surgeons hungry. The interaction between the cardiologist and the cardiac surgeon has veered erratically between cooperation and competition over the years as technologies have changed. This complicated relationship is more than vaguely reminiscent of the relationship between large-cat species, such as lions and cheetahs, and dog species, like the hyenas and jackals, on the African veldt.

We adopted a new dog within months of the deaths of Chaos and Mayhem—a hybrid between a poodle and a golden retriever, popularly and somewhat awkwardly called a Goldendoodle. The Goldendoodle derives its ancestry from two different breeds of the retriever family, and, while not yet sanctioned by kennel clubs, it has become quite popular. Goldendoodles are "lovable, well-mannered, intelligent dogs with a great charm...they enjoy pleasing their masters...love to swim, and...have little, if any, guarding instincts."[10]

Curiously, dog and doctor species both have evolved to address the diseases of Western society. Doodles are touted as being hypoallergenic and an attractive alternative for owners who like the disposition of the golden retriever but want a dog that sheds less hair, both of which are desirable to owners who like a clean and allergen-free home. However, we've come to find out that allergies and asthma are actually preventable diseases of the modern Western world, and some researchers attribute the increase in the incidence of these diseases since the 1960s to our increasingly hygienic, germ-free childhoods.

An increasingly accepted theory has it that the immune systems of our children are not adequately challenged in our spanking-clean homes, and allergies result from the consequently incomplete development of their immune systems. We know that the immune system actually *needs* exposure to germs to learn the difference between "self" and "non-self." In fact, Swedish kids who grow up on farms have fewer allergies than their city counterparts who grow up on the sterile, sleek surfaces of Scandinavian kitchen floors.[11] So, when we should be encouraging our kids to grow up like little cave trolls, instead we sterilize our homes with Lysol, breed hypoallergenic dogs, like goldendoodles, and then send the children to specialists in "Allergy, Asthma and Immunology" for inhalers and desensitization shots. Similarly, we feed our children calorie-rich soda and fruit juice, sugary cereals and salty chips, thereby ending up raising a generation of obese adults who need the services of "bariatricians."

The Flexner Report produced what ecologists would probably call a *mass extinction.* In response to its recommendations, half of the medical schools in the country closed, and the proprietary, for-profit model of medical education became extinct more or less immediately. Viewed from one vantage, this was a catastrophic die-off—it was as if medical education had been struck by a comet. Today, however, we regard the dramatic results of the Flexner Report as a beginning—the birth of modern scientific medicine.

Within a very few years of the report, the rapid proliferation of medical specialties began. Ecologists call this explosive diversification after a major environmental stress *adaptive radiation,* which is defined as "rapid evolutionary radiation characterized by an increase in the morphological and ecological diversity of a single, rapidly diversifying lineage."[12] In adaptive radiation, phenotypes change in response to the environment by developing new and useful traits. Classic examples are the replacement of dinosaurs by mammals and the evolution of different finch species with a variety of beaks in the Galapagos Islands—finches being a species that Charles Darwin studied extensively.

The Galapagos finches diversified as they migrated from the mainland to one isolated ecosystem, an island like the ones studied by E. O. Wilson, and then to more distant islands with different food sources. Some finches evolved long, pointy beaks, which are good for catching and eating insects. Others developed a broad, stout beak designed to crush seeds. A third species developed a blunt beak that allowed it to tear vegetation. These adaptations arose because the food sources differed on each of the islands colonized by the finches, as the ecosystems varied. The island ecological niche turns out to be a useful metaphor for examining a puzzling thing about medical care in today's sub-specialized hospitals: the wide variation in practice patterns and medical costs among hospitals.

In a June 2009 article in the *New Yorker* magazine, Atul Gawande, a physician and medical writer, analyzed the medical costs in McAllen, Texas, "the most expensive town in the most expensive country for health care in the world."[13] He learned that compared to almost anywhere else in the United States, McAllen patients got more diagnostic testing, hospital treatment, surgery and home care. In fact, McAllen's Medicare costs were more than twice that of the Mayo Clinic on a per-enrollee basis—and Mayo has outstanding outcomes, while McAllen hospitals' outcomes were average at best. Perhaps most interesting, the health-care providers in McAllen were oblivious to their outlier status. It's as if they were living on one island, and their counterparts at Mayo were on a different one.

The doctors from the McAllen medical island referred patients back and forth among specialists. Their notes probably read like this: "Dr. Cardiologist, please evaluate Mrs. Smith's heart before I take out her gall bladder." And they got lots of tests: "In anticipation of your consultation, I took the liberty of ordering a cardiac ultrasound and stress test for Mrs. Smith as per your usual...." Each referral and test increased cost. They provided what amounted to fat medical care in McAllen. In fact McAllen was like a medical Samoa, an island where the obesity rate is over 75 percent.

At Mayo, on the other hand, medical care is lean. It's the medical New Guinea, an island where tribes practice subsistence farming. At Mayo, they practice subsistence medicine, and there's no excess fat. The cultures of these two medical islands, Mayo and McAllen, are distinctly different. McAllen's culture is the traditional "fee-for-service" model, where the doctor gets a fee for each service she provides—more services, more fees. Fee-for-service reimbursement is the model preferred by the American Medical Association, but at Mayo everyone is on a salary, and there are no rewards for greater services. Coincidentally or not, this has resulted in lean, high-quality medical care. We'll explore the tension between fee-for-service medicine and the salaried model in greater detail in the next chapter, which looks at the history of the Kaiser health plan.

The lack of a single-payer system and, as we'll see, the provinciality of medical records and data in the United States has permitted the development of thousands of heterogeneous islands of medical behavior, ranging from profit-oriented specialty hospitals to large nonprofit health systems with a significant burden of unreimbursed care. Gawande's comparative observations about the costs at McAllen and Mayo are possible now because we've begun to analyze large medical databases showing cost- and quality-outlier islands, bad and good.

If asked, the vast majority of health-care providers would still have no idea where they lie on the cost/quality scale—but they'd naturally assume they were above average. In fact, Gawande describes a conversation he had with one McAllen hospital CEO, held "around one end of a yacht length table," who defended the above-average costs of his doctors, saying that they "are providing necessary, essential healthcare—we don't invent patients."[14] Reading between the lines, one senses the profound mutual incomprehension of the two parties to this conversation.

Gawande's piece was written at the end of a "Fat Era," in which banks got fat, people got fat and even our pets got fat. The Fat Era is being followed by a "Lean Era"—the Great Recession. Pets and people have been put on forced diets. So were banks and hospitals—the latter in large part because of increases in unemployed and therefore uninsured patients. Nobody knows what form the future will take in medicine, but we can be pretty certain that the new medicine will be leaner and more efficient and that its practitioners will evolve and adapt to the times. In other words, we're about to see new species of doctors and other medical providers with new skill sets.

One of the most frequent complaints my friends make about their medical care, often in an outraged tone of voice, is about the bills they get. If they have even a small surgery, for example, they get a bill from the hospital and separate ones from the surgeon and the anesthesiologist. The latter are what we in the trade call *pro-fees,* which is short for *professional fees*—the fees-for-service described in Gawande's *New Yorker* article about medical costs in McAllen, Texas. While the term professional fee sounds modern, it's actually a way medical care has been paid for since the dawn of medicine. A century ago, the doctor might deliver your baby or pull your tooth in return for whatever it was that *you* produced, perhaps flour, bacon or dry goods. The professional fee back then might even have been a piglet. Now, of course, most of us have medical insurance, and there's no palpable or direct exchange of goods—the insurance company pays the bills and, if you work, your employer pays for the insurance.

Some refer to the fee-for-service model as an "eat what you kill" approach, which, while awkward for a variety of reasons, is an apt description of the way things work in the for-profit medical world. A doctor who sees lots of patients, or bills for lots of services, eats well…sometimes very well. Health systems court successful doctors like these, because the hospital gets a piece of the action as well.

In a lot of ways, the ecology of the for-profit medical world is analogous to the African veldt, with its very transparent food chain. On the savannah, an apex-predator like a lion brings down a game animal and eats; then a second group of smaller scavenger-predators like the jackal, hyena and vulture move in to get some of the better leavings. Eventually, after several waves of diners, the carcass is nibbled clean and all that's left is the buzzing of the flies and the dung beetles scurrying around under the hot sun.

The apex-predator equivalents in today's medical food chain are typically "rainmakers" in the more profitable specialties like orthopedics and neurosurgery. Anesthesiologists, radiologists, pathologists, respiratory therapists and hospital administrators wait further down in the food chain to get their bite of the carcass. At the bottom, smiling from billboards and city buses, personal injury lawyers toil under that same hot sun.

The fee-for-service model has been tweaked repeatedly in various recent efforts to control medical costs over the past several decades, but the optimal financial strategy for a health-care delivery organization has always been some variant of "admit more patients with well-reimbursed surgical conditions." Physician-owned bariatric and cardiac hospitals, like in McAllen, are structured around these lucrative specialties and exemplify this strategy.

These hospitals were created to take advantage of what some have described as a loophole in laws that had been designed to prevent a physician from referring business to himself—and that loophole effectively acts as a kind of ecological niche. The loophole permits business-minded doctors to reroute "profitable" patients from general multi-specialty hospitals to specialty hospitals in which the doctors hold an interest (and, of course, cannibalize the profits of the source institution in the process). The doctor-owner thus gets the professional fees for his own work as well as a second bite of the apple from the specialty hospital's profits. This is Darwinism at work in medicine—the strong wresting resources from the weak.

In a physician-owned specialty hospital, doctors obviously are in charge, which is just the way they want it. A standard health-care organization, however, is run by professional hospital administrators who try to balance the needs of the various players in the organization in meeting the hospital's mission, but Darwin's laws favoring the strong are at work here as well. In order to illustrate how the strong prevail in a typical, non-specialty hospital, let's imagine the internal budgetary deliberations in a profitable, well-run community hospital somewhere in America called Memorial General Hospital.

Our imaginary CEO is Hiram Stark, a 60-ish, patrician gentleman with piercing blue eyes and the lean body of a runner. The CFO is Geraldine Pinch, a crisp 40-year-old with short, straight brown hair wearing stainless-steel reading glasses on a lanyard. Dr. Fred Phudge is president of the medical staff; he's a short, balding 50-year-old rheumatologist who weighs 20 pounds more than he'd like to. Phudge was elected to his position because he'd never offended anyone during his 20 years at the hospital.

Up for consideration at today's meeting are three capital requests for the next fiscal year. The first is the Utistop computer system requested by Dr. Phineas Pimpole, the hospital infection control officer. It uses sophisticated computer algorithms to flag patients at risk for hospital-acquired infections like pneumonia or urinary tract infections. Dr. Melvin Meningus, a busy neurosurgeon on staff, has demanded the purchase of a CranioMorpher Laser, noting that Central across town just got one, and he needs to keep up, "Goddammit!" Finally, Dr. Stan Sternem, the hospital's cardiac surgeon, says he needs a CoronoRooter to enhance the hospital's highly profitable cardiac surgical service line. None of these three gentlemen will be at the budgetary meeting. The hospital's marketing pitch is: "Just imagine!—the latest in High-Tech medical services with the Personal touch of a Community Hospital."

The dollar amounts for the three requests are all roughly equivalent, but the hospital can only afford to approve one of them—hence the ad hoc meeting of our group.

Stark already knows which option he's going to approve, but likes to give the appearance of building consensus. He asks, "Fred, what do you think about this Utistop system? I don't know much about it."

Dr. Phudge does not like to inch out on a limb on his own and certainly doesn't like being pushed out there, but timidly offers in response, "Well, Hiram, we just had an outbreak of *E. coli* bacterial urinary infections on the surgical ward, and I think it might be useful to have some way to track and maybe prevent these problems going forward. Dr. Pimpole is pretty concerned because the *E. coli* is resistant to most antibiotics, and our bladder infection rate is already higher than the national average."

Stark looks over to his CFO and says, "Pinch?"

She squares up the papers in front of her, and pushes down the reading glasses before looking over them at the two men. Tightening her lips and drawing a long, slow breath in through her nose, she responds: "Well, as you both know, I see investment in IT as adding cost and nothing to the bottom line. Both Dr. Meningus and Dr. Sternem bring in a lot of patients, and we can't afford to offend them. They're competing in a tough market.... And, by the way, we *do* get paid extra to take care of those patients with the bladder infections."

Stark smiles imperceptibly and says, "Well, that settles it. We'll get the CoronoRooter. Meningus and the infection control folks can resubmit next year."

Phudge pops a breath mint into his mouth and looks away from Pinch who, in turn, makes a neat check mark next to the winner before lining out the losers with her neatly sharpened, number-2 Ticonderoga pencil.

In the old-fashioned fee-for-service environment, medical rainmakers like Meningus and Sternem have an evolutionary advantage over poor Phineas Pimpole, the infection control officer, because under traditional payment schemes, the hospital makes more when Meningus and Sternem admit more patients *and* it makes more even if patients develop complications. So it wouldn't pay to put money into a system like the one advocated by Pimpole, which is designed to decrease reimbursable infections. But a new era is coming.

As the *New England Journal* put it, sort of succinctly, in a 2009 editorial: "Rising health care costs and an economic downturn have intensified the pressure for cost savings, even as the new presidential administration is seeking to broaden access to insurance coverage. There are probably just two ways to resolve these tensions: providers must be paid less for transactions under fee for service, or they must be paid differently."[15]

The way physicians and health-care organizations will be paid in the future will be based to a much greater degree than in the past on the *quality* of their work—a shift to what is known in the trade as *pay-for-performance* payment reform. As hard as it is to believe, until recently we've never kept close track of physician or hospital outcomes, or costs for that matter, in any meaningful way. So we haven't had an accurate way of measuring performance, much less rewarding it when it is good. One way of understanding the difference between fee-for-service and pay-for-performance is to reimagine the budgetary discussions at Memorial General in the coming era—when good results *do* make a positive difference to the hospital bottom line, and poor performance costs. And let's add a little background information that I didn't give you before.

It turns out that Dr. Stan Sternem has secrets. Earlier in his career, Stan was a really good surgeon. He trained at a top-notch program and was a great recruit for Memorial General. Over a period of years, he's built up quite a referral base. Cardiologists from a hundred-mile radius send him patients by land, and more recently, by helicopter, to have their heart surgery. But Stan's not the man he used to be. He's developed bipolar disorder, or what is more commonly called manic-depression, and he swings between up and down periods. His marriage is on the rocks, partly because of his behavior, partly because he's never at home. In fact, things have gotten so uneven that he's taken on a junior partner to help him get through his caseload and who's begun to do more and more of the work.

Sternem's team of doctors and nurses find him trying to work with, and morale has deteriorated. So have their results. His patients have more infections, longer stays and more operative complications. In fact, two patients in the past year have had to go back to the operating room to have surgical sponges removed. But the referrals keep coming, which is a curious thing about medicine. Because of the historical lack of concurrent and reliable data about the quality of a doctor's work, his reputation is disproportion-ately important—and a good reputation sometimes lasts long even after it's no longer merited. The interesting consequence is that in a fee-for-service environment, or ecosystem, as long as Sternem keeps bringing patients into the hospital, he'll continue to be a valued, albeit difficult to handle, asset for the hospital. That's why Geraldine Pinch went to bat for him at the budget table in our first scenario. Let's see how the same conversation might go in the new pay-for-*performance* ecosystem.

Stark, Pinch and Phudge are still sitting around the table. The furniture in the board room doesn't smell of furniture polish anymore; it's cracked and scuffed and the seats of the chairs are a little frayed. Phudge has gotten a personal trainer and has slimmed down to his fighting weight. As if to com-pensate, Stark has put on a little gut. Just as before, Stark turns to Phudge and says, "Fred, what do you think about this Utistop system? I don't know much about it."

This Fred is slim and feistier. He answers, "Hiram, we *need* that sys-tem, goddammit. Our hospital infections are out of control, and our out-comes are plummeting on the very public Hospital Compare website. Medicare doesn't pay us a cent for the patients who get infected anymore, and we'd see the return on investment in less than a year without any problem!"

Stark looks over to his CFO and says, "Pinch?"

She's in a difficult position—because *her* secret is that she and Sternem once had a little thing going on. And he, in his manic way, has lobbied her ceaselessly over the past few weeks for the CoronoRooter. She squares up the papers in front of her and peers pointedly at them through her reading glasses. With a quick breath, as if before a plunge, she says: "Well, I think we might have already put enough into IT this past year. Both Dr. Meningus and Dr. Sternem bring in a lot of patients and, in my opinion, we can't afford to offend them. They're competing in a tough market."

Stark smiles slightly, and says, "Well, Geraldine, Sternem's got a couple of big lawsuits pending, and he may not be around much longer. I agree with Fred. We have to keep our numbers up on the quality front. Let's go with the Utistop system."

Phudge cracks his knuckles and looks over at Pinch, who is studiously cleaning some imperceptible debris from under a painted fingernail with her sharpest number-2 Ticonderoga pencil.

Just as in the real world, there will be winners and losers as the ecology changes. The rest of the book is about medicine's new practitioners: who they will be, what they will do, the tools they will use and what that will mean for us as patients. Just as today's children seem born with computer skills their parents will never achieve, tomorrow's doctors will use those same skills in the practice of medicine in ways we can't yet imagine. Children who grew up playing Quake and Doom will learn how to practice medicine in simulated medical environments not too different from those fantasy computer games. The next generation of doctors may practice in virtual worlds as well, where medical information is mapped onto the real world in some form of heads-up display. Automated medical instruments, like cockpit autopilots, will control machines that currently require constant attention from doctors, nurses and respiratory therapists. Today's printed medical journals will become tomorrow's websites, and the cycle of medical discovery to publication to implementation will shorten commensurately.

From the medical consumer's standpoint, a generation of patients who grew up with Google, eBay and Wikipedia will soon have access to comparably comprehensive, current information about medicine and its practitioners. They'll be able to find best-performing doctors and hospitals in the same way they can now shop for best-buy electronics and credit card rates. The successful practitioner and medical systems of the future will be the ones that adapt best to the new patient, who was raised on universal information and immediate gratification.

CHAPTER 8

SUCH WASTE IS TRAGIC

Sarah Stone is 45. She is a physician assistant who worked for years at a mid-sized community hospital, with a cardiac surgeon in an active practice. Her job was to scrub in during heart operations and harvest the long *saphenous* vein (the word derives its roots from Greek and Arabic and means "hidden"); it runs along the inside of each leg from the foot to the groin and is used as the piping for coronary artery bypass grafting. She would carefully clip the feeder vessels that drained into the vein, and then draw a blue stripe down the length of the vessel so the surgeon could see if it was twisted while it was being sewn in. Sarah would then hand the worm-like vein to the doctor, who would cut it into segments which were then used to bypass blood flow around blocked coronary vessels. At the end of her day, Sarah would round on post-op patients in the intensive care unit with the heart surgeon, and she'd become quite adept at handling the routine critical-care problems with blood pressure and breathing that developed in the immediate hours after surgery. However, the surgeon retired a year ago, and while she had filled in part-time at the hospital since then, Sarah had come to treasure her free time during the day, which she could spend with her children or, better yet, on herself. But she needed to work.

Rajeesh Desai is 33 and Indian. He went to medical school in Mumbai and practiced there as a general surgeon for two years but eventually decided he wanted to come to the United States. Because of the requirements of American medical licensure, Raj needed to start over and complete a new residency in the states in order to be eligible for an unrestricted licensure to practice medicine—despite the fact that he had been a practicing physician in his home country. Desai eventually obtained a spot in what's called the *scramble*, wherein unmatched residency applicants and residencies with unfilled spots try to pair up in a giant, one-day game of musical chairs held every year on March 16. By then, the bulk of the spots have already been filled during the traditional match, which is designed to give residents and residencies the best chance of getting their highest ranked choices. Married with a wife and a 2-year-old boy, Desai needs to work while awaiting the beginning of a fellowship.

Frank Delacourt is 58, and a former surgeon from Ohio with degenerative arthritis of both hips—he is unable to stand for the prolonged periods required of the operations he's trained to perform. He has two children from a second marriage who are about to enter college, and his savings are insufficient to cover the tuition. He has a greenhouse in his backyard where he cultivates orchids as a hobby. He's also a gourmet cook. He needs to work.

None of these skilled health-care professionals is able to practice independently for different reasons, and yet each has a wealth of experience and a desire to work. A decade ago, it would have been difficult for them to find the kind of job that suited their needs. Now they all work at night as what are called *nocturnalists*—nighttime practitioners.

Regional General Hospital, another imaginary hospital like the one run by Stark, Pinch and Phudge, is a 400-bed urban facility affiliated with a major academic medical school. Its health-care mission is bifurcated. On the one hand, it serves a large indigent population that suffers from the health-care problems typical of that group: hypertension, diabetes and infectious diseases like HIV. This kind of care is, at best, a break-even proposition for Regional General, albeit critical to the community. However, the hospital also has several top-notch surgeons and medical specialists; and it acts as a regional transfer center for patients with heart and lung disease. The cardiologists accept referrals of acute cardiac patients from a hundred-mile radius, flying them in on heart-rescue helicopter flights that run day and night.

The medical and surgical procedures required by these heart patients—such as cardiac angiography, heart vessel stents and open-heart surgery—are very profitable for the hospital, and it has invested a good deal of money in state-of-the-art cardiac catheterization labs, operating rooms and intensive care units. As these "product lines" expanded, the hospital's administration realized it would need to open additional intensive care beds and staff them with more nurses and doctors. It was at this time that they ran into an unexpected problem.

Nursing supply has waxed and waned periodically over the decades in most countries, competing with other employment options for young men and women entering the workforce. But nursing is a rewarding career, relatively recession-proof, and it offers a gateway to a wide range of other options down the road. It isn't that difficult to hire new nurses at thriving hospitals like Regional General. It wasn't even that difficult to hire a team of intensive care specialists for the new surgical ICU that was built as part of the expansion in critical care beds; the hospital worked with one of the academic departments from the affiliated medical school to bring in a new team of these relatively scarce specialists.

The problem turned up when it came time to staff the new unit with so-called *mid-level providers,* the "house doctors" who are physically stationed in the hospital round the clock. Before the advent of work-hour limitations, the universal answer to *all* mid-level physician staffing requirements at any academically affiliated hospital was the same: use the residents who constitute the house staff.

Residents were like duct tape or chewing gum: they could be used to fill almost any need, they could be stretched to cover any gap, or they could be stuffed into any hole. If you needed more coverage, you could (a) hire more residents, (b) have the residents cover more patients and/or (c) change their call schedule from, say, every third to every other night, or (d) all of the above. No worries—instant workforce expansion. But after an infamous medical case from the mid-1980s that I'll describe in the next chapter, residents were limited by strict "hours of duty" rules, and new workers were needed to fill the void. Suddenly there was a desperate need for mid-level providers—apprentices—for hire, particularly at night when there were fewer staff doctors around.

Anticipating this need, nursing schools had revved up their graduate programs for nurse practitioners, and physician assistant programs proliferated. But the problem was that many of the people who went into these programs did so specifically to get away from the nighttime shift work that is a routine part of the regular nurse's job. What became increasingly apparent in the years following the institution of duty-hour limitations was a new need for mid-level or experienced health-care providers who were willing to work at night to fill in the gaps that used to be filled by residents—that is, to be the night watchmen. In effect, the void created by duty-hour restrictions created a sort of ecological niche or opportunity for a nocturnal species of health-care provider.

As we saw earlier, medicine underwent a period of explosive proliferation following the Flexner Report in the first decade of the twentieth century. New specialties developed, each of which began with a few pioneers, who trained acolytes, which spawned new residencies; and new residencies meant more workers. It was a time of plenty. But things began to change in the late 1980s.

As medical costs began to balloon in the 1970s, the U.S. government started to pay attention and began to study ways to check the growth in medicine that it had previously encouraged. Prior to that time, Medicare had paid whatever a hospital charged for a patient's stay; but by the 1980s, prodded in part by general economic concerns, Congress and the Reagan administration recognized that Medicare would be insolvent in the near future if there wasn't some fundamental change in the way they did business. So they set out to study alternatives.

The government looked at a number of potential solutions, but the one that eventually won out flipped the balance of power between the payer and the payee like a black-belt judo move. Rather than the government continuing to pay whatever it was charged by hospitals, essentially guaranteeing continuous growth and leaving the industry with the upper hand, come 1983, Medicare instituted a prospective payment scheme in which it set a reimbursement rate based on the patient's diagnosis; and it paid ahead of time, explicitly putting a cap on the amount the hospital was paid to care for a specific type of patient. From then forward, rates were reset every year, and financial control shifted to the government after this reversal of power.

The institution of what was called *diagnosis-related group (DRG)–based reimbursement* represented the first of what went on to become a seemingly endless series of supply-side constraints on medicine's previously inexorable expansion. Resident work-hour restrictions were another. Managed care, a term used to describe a combination of measures including explicit controls on costly interventions and intensive management of high-cost cases, was yet a third. And as with any ecosystem under stress, medicine responded to these new resource constraints with adaptations of its own.

As I've described in the last chapter, medical specialties and sub-specialties historically branched off from a main discipline as new medical knowledge developed in a new area. However, in 1996, a *New England Journal* opinion piece described the first of a new breed of specialties that developed explicitly in response to the changes in the way doctors worked. The authors said: "We anticipate the rapid growth of a new breed of physicians we call hospitalists—specialists in inpatient medicine—who will be responsible for managing the care of hospitalized patients in the same way that primary care physicians are responsible for managing the care of outpatients."[1] They went on to elaborate:

> We believe the hospitalist specialty will burgeon for several reasons. First, because of cost pressures, managed-care organizations will reward professionals who can provide efficient care. In the outpatient setting, the premium on efficiency requires that the physician provide care for a large panel of patients and be available in the office to see them promptly as required. There is no greater barrier to efficiency in outpatient care than the need to go across the street (or even worse, across town) to the hospital to see an unpredictable number of inpatients, sometimes several times a day. There are parallel pressures for efficiency in the hospital. Since the inpatient setting involves the most intensive use of resources, it is the place where the ability to respond quickly to changes in a patient's condition and to use resources judiciously will be most highly valued. This should prove to be the hospitalists' forte.

The authors, Bob Wachter and Lee Goldman, proved to be spot-on with their predictions. The hospitalist model grew so rapidly over the succeeding decade that what subsequently became the Society of Hospital Medicine now has roughly 10,000 members. While the original hospitalists were all internists, specializing in the care of the adult hospitalized patient, there are now pediatric, obstetric and family-practice equivalents.

By 1996, the development of a new specialty was certainly not that novel; medicine had been on a specialization binge for decades. What *was* interesting about this new hospitalist specialty, however, was the impetus for its development. As Wachter and Goldman note in their description, "cost pressures" and the "premium on efficiency" inherent in managed care changed the way primary care physicians practiced in the latter half of the 1990s.

In the previous era, an internist would see patients in her office and simultaneously direct the care of those patients if they were hospitalized, sometimes moving back and forth repeatedly between the two venues on a given day. In fact, this is the primary reason that medical office buildings have historically been built next to hospitals—so that the doctors would have only a short walk to get to the hospital to see their inpatients. In that era, as depicted on shows like *Marcus Welby, M.D.*, it was dogma that the same doctor directed his patient's care through periods of health and illness, or, as Wachter and Goldman put it in their article:

> Ideally, the primary care physician would provide all aspects of care, ranging from preventive care to the care of critically ill hospitalized patients. This approach, argued the purists, would result in medical care that was more holistic, less fragmented, and less expensive. To its proponents, the notion was so attractive—the general internist admits the patient to the hospital, directs the inpatient workup, and arranges for a seamless transition back to the outpatient setting— that questioning it would have seemed sacrilegious merely a few years ago.

The fact of the matter was that, by 1996, the Welby era was over, and the formal coining of the term *hospitalist* was analogous to the development of the expression *piecework* during the Industrial Revolution. Both are terms specific to an industry that holds clues about what was going on in the industry at the time the term was coined. The latter actually has its origins in the craft guilds: a Master would assign the construction of parts—pieces—of a whole work to individual apprentices. Eli Whitney is credited with the development of an assembly process by which piece workers would make many exact copies of a single equipment part, like a gear, using a machine tool, like a lathe. The various component parts from geographically dispersed piece workers would then be connected into a whole product at some central location. Whitney invented a musket that was assembled in this fashion from pieces like locks, stocks and barrels.

The next logical step in improving the efficiency of machine construction was the development of assembly lines, with all of the piece workers lined up together along a conveyor belt as they assembled a final product in sequence from its constituent parts—a process patented by Ransom Olds and later refined by the Ford Motor Company. In an interesting historical footnote, one of Ford's assembly-line collaborators was actually inspired by the efficiency with which animals were funneled into the front ends of Chicago's slaughterhouses of the era and progressively *dis*assembled into meat, piece by piece, where each butcher along the disassembly line was responsible for a specific cut. Regardless of whether the task was assembly or disassembly, the key to the efficiency of such a line is the fact that the worker stays put, in one place, with the work coming to him.

The unstated, but obvious, subtext to the Wachter-Goldman *New England Journal* editorial was their observation that the sundowning of the fee-for-service reimbursement model would dramatically increase pressure on the average office-based practitioner to stay put, like an assembly-line worker, as patients marched through the examination rooms in a long, gray line—often as many as 25 to 35 per day.

The days of the free-range, Marcus Welby-esque internist had passed, their editorial was saying. The modern internist would be much more like a cooped chicken or a penned calf: confined to a single location with a piped-in supply of basic requirements like patients, nurses, medical records and pens. In the modern era, it would no longer be practical, desirable or even feasible to simultaneously manage an office practice and a group of hospitalized inpatients.

The hospitalist editorial was published in one of the most widely read medical periodicals in the world, and it got a lot of attention among physicians when it first came out, because the concept initially seemed so bizarre to many of us. In the past, doctors had *always* made rounds, going wherever they needed to see their patients. As Abraham Flexner had put it in 1910, "*ambulando discimus.*" We learned by going about.

In fact, the very name chosen for the new specialty was aberrant. Medical specialties in the past had always either identified "the thing that the doctor did," like radiology, pathology or anesthesiology, or the "population the doctor cared for," like pediatrics or geriatrics. Never before had a medical specialty been named after the *location* of the care. The term *hospitalist* was like the term *doorman*—more descriptive of where the worker worked than what he did, and the new name subliminally suggested that something weird was happening in medicine. Wachter and Goldman were describing a new type of doctor who was assigned to cover a physical space and the patients who passed through it, rather than what "normal" doctors did, which was to follow patients as they moved from office to hospital and back, through the course of each patient's lifetime.

The basketball coach of the Newton High School in Kansas between 1914 and 1945 was a man named Frank Lindley. Lindley was an early basketball theorist and wrote books on the topic. During his three decades as a coach, his teams amassed a 594–118 record, won ten state titles and came in second seven times. In other words, over a 30-year stretch, without the ability to recruit (because it was a public high school), Lindley's teams came in first or second in the state more than half of the time.

One of the innovations with which Lindley is credited is the zone defense, which was completely revolutionary in its time and contributed to his teams' dominance. Lindley's new zone-coverage scheme was a radical departure from the man-to-man defense that was standard prior to that time. In man-to-man, the coach tells each of his players which guy he's covering. Lindley told each of his players what portion of the basketball court he was covering—which *space* was his. One player might be told to cover opposing players who enter the lane, which is the space under the basket; another, one of the flanking positions.

There are lots of situations in basketball, as well as in other sports, in which zone has advantages over man-to-man coverage. For example, zone coverage is one way for a team to neutralize single-player mismatches in which a guard or a forward on the offensive team is too fast or too tall for any one of the individuals who might be assigned to cover him in a "man" scheme. Because it often takes time and patience to break down and score against a zone defense, these schemes are also used to slow down the pace of a game, allowing a team to sit on a lead.

A significant and related advantage of this geographically oriented defensive scheme, and one that makes it increasingly relevant to medical care, is the fact that defensive players can get some rest in a zone. As with basketball, the pace of medicine seems to have sped up dramatically over the past decade or two; the doctor just doesn't have time to take an afternoon off every week for a game of golf anymore. Today's doctors are working harder to stay in one place.

Compared to Marcus Welby, who might have seen eight to ten office patients a day, followed by rounds in the hospital, a modern office-based practitioner sees about 25. In an eight-hour day, with no lunch break, that means 19 minutes per patient. Some of those patients will be return visits and may not take that long. However, others will be brand new to the doctor, with complicated past medical records, and they need time to tell their story. The doctor also has to do an examination, write prescriptions and document the encounter in the medical record.

The growing emphasis on medical office throughput is what prompted Wachter and Goldman to write: "We believe the hospitalist specialty will burgeon for several reasons. First, because of cost pressures, managed-care organizations will reward professionals who can provide efficient care. In the outpatient setting, the premium on efficiency requires that the physician provide care for a large panel of patients and be available in the office to see them promptly as required." This was their nice way of saying that the medical office was becoming industrialized, which is not surprising when one understands the historical roots of managed care and the critical differences between it and the competing fee-for-service model preferred by organized medicine through much of the twentieth century.

In 1933, the world was in the midst of the Great Depression. Much as it has done recently, the United States government undertook big public works projects to buttress employment. One such project was the construction of an aqueduct designed to carry water from Lake Havasu in Arizona to Southern California.

The lake is a giant reservoir on the Colorado River behind the Parker Dam, and its waters are siphoned off and carried across 150 miles of the Mojave Desert, around a series of small mountain ranges, through a 13-mile-long tunnel in the San Jacinto Mountains and thence to its coastal destinations. Absent this water supply, the explosive growth of Southern California would not have been possible. At the peak of construction, the project employed nearly 30,000 workers who were subject to all of the illnesses and injuries inherent in extremely challenging construction of what would eventually be named one of the engineering marvels of the modern world. Needless to say, there weren't hospitals in the middle of the desert equipped to handle this new, but temporary, supply of patients.

Recognizing an opportunity, a young surgeon fresh out of his residency at Los Angeles County Hospital borrowed $2,500 from his father and built what he subsequently named Contractor's General Hospital, a 12-bed facility at a work camp along the course of the aqueduct. Dr. Sidney

Garfield built and furnished the building with equipment and supplies that came, like the air-conditioner he was loaned by General Electric, "on spec." Garfield was the son of Russian immigrants and had trained at the University of Iowa as well as in Chicago and Los Angeles. He was an idealistic and enthusiastic young man with modern ideas about how a hospital should look and work.

Contractor's General Hospital was positioned at the eastern end of a tunnel blasted through the Eagle Mountains, which formed a north-south obstacle to the path of the east-west aqueduct. Tunnel construction proceeded around the clock and involved dangerous work with explosives and big chunks of rock.

Garfield saw his role in the provision of definitive care to patients where possible and stabilization for transport to more sophisticated and well-equipped Los Angeles hospitals in more critically ill cases. Within months of the hospital's opening, Garfield was treating an active population of sick and injured construction workers. Unfortunately, he was also broke, because the workers' insurer, the Industrial Indemnity Exchange, failed to pay his bills on time, and he refused to turn away patients who couldn't afford to pay. Garfield got everything right—he had a new hospital, had plenty of patients, and was needed and respected—except for the payment model, which relied on the traditional fee-for-service paradigm. He would, in all likelihood, have ended up packing up and moving to a larger metropolitan hospital were it not for support from an unexpected source.

The Industrial Indemnity Exchange was not like today's large medical insurers, who have no interest in the success or failure of an individual physician. The exchange was actually an insurance consortium formed by the aqueduct's construction contractors to handle their workers' injury compensation claims. And while it had been slow to pay claims, the company had been formed by contractors who had every interest in the success of Dr. Garfield's little hospital that kept their employees healthy enough to work around the clock on the Eagle Mountain tunnel.

Two of Industrial Indemnity's executives, one of whom had been an engineer in a "previous life," eventually came to young Dr. Garfield with a proposal that quickly improved the finances of Contractor's General. The approach they settled on in that dusty little town in a California desert eventually spawned what is now one of the largest health-care organizations in the world.

Alonzo Ordway and Harold Hatch, who was an engineer turned insurance agent, suggested a way to reengineer the financial arrangement between Garfield and the company. The insurance company would *prospectively* pay 17.5 percent of the industrial premium directly to Garfield, or $1.50 per worker per month, to cover work-related injuries, and the worker would sign up for additional, nonindustrial coverage through a voluntary, nickel-a-day payroll deduction.

With these front-loaded payments, Garfield was able to turn the finances of the hospital around and eventually found he could move from crisis management to a more preventative focus on safety. In contrasting the traditional fee-for-service, crisis management approach with this new prepaid health-care arrangement, Garfield later said: "To the private physician, the sick person is an asset. To us, the sick person is a liability. We'd go bankrupt if we didn't keep most of our members well most of the time."

By the time the aqueduct had been completed, Garfield was running a group of ten doctors with the necessary support staff at three hospitals. His debts were gone and he was actually in the black by about $150,000 (a not-insignificant sum at that time). But when the construction workers moved on, so, too, did his business, so Garfield returned to Los Angeles for further medical training with the eventual intent of entering private practice. But Hatch and Ordway hadn't forgotten him. Their primary employer was a large construction company formed decades earlier by another classic self-made man who had dropped out of school, bored already at the age of 13.

Like Garfield, Henry Kaiser was born the son of immigrants—Germans in his case—in upstate New York. He knocked about in a series of jobs in a dry-goods store and photography shop, among others, in his teen years and eventually fell in love with a young woman from a higher socioeconomic class, whose father insisted he prove himself before proposing marriage. Kaiser headed west on a train to Spokane, Washington, where he eventually found work, bought a house and settled with his bride, Bess—having won the approval of her family.

Kaiser recognized that the increasing popularity of cars and the absence of good roads in the Northwest presented an opportunity, and he got into the business of paving roads. He was a visionary, extremely hardworking and an optimist. Within a few years the Kaisers had moved south to Oakland and moved beyond roads to larger construction projects around the United States and as far away as Cuba.

The big public works ventures during the Great Depression included highways, aqueducts and dams. Kaiser's company, working with an engineering firm named Bechtel, put together a consortium to build the Hoover Dam. Kaiser Construction went on to play a role in building the Colorado River Aqueduct, the Bonneville Dam and the Grand Coulee Dam—both of the latter on the Columbia River. As cement was a key ingredient in construction, Kaiser had occasion to visit many limestone quarries and eventually built a cement plant on Black Mountain near what is now a city named Cupertino. The Ria Permanente or "permanent creek" was a stream that ran by the plant.

Henry and Bess appreciated the reliability of this small but perpetual water source during California's dry seasons that lasted so many months of each year. Permanente became a watchword for the couple that they subsequently acknowledged with the formation of Kaiser Permanente, the now-giant health maintenance organization. But that wouldn't happen until 1942, well after Henry Kaiser and Sidney Garfield had what would become a fateful meeting in the late 1930s. These two remarkable visionaries, born 25 years apart, began a professional working relationship that turned into a friendship—one that ultimately became almost incestuous.

In 1938, Garfield was back in Los Angeles preparing for private practice when he was contacted by Hatch and Ordway, the two Industrial Indemnity insurance agents, who were now working with the Kaiser company on the Grand Coulee Dam. They arranged a meeting between Garfield and Edgar Kaiser, Henry's son, who was running the Grand Coulee project, and Edgar persuaded Garfield to reproduce his successful medical model from the aqueduct at the dam. Garfield bought a decrepit hospital overlooking the dam site and renovated its two-story wood-frame building. The new Mason City Hospital had 75 beds and employed 8 physicians as well as 51 support staff. It was also a very busy enterprise, providing nearly 4,000 treatments per month.[2]

Garfield's business model evolved quickly at Grand Coulee, which remains the largest cement structure in the world and was designed to generate electricity for the Pacific Northwest. Unlike workers on the aqueduct, many of the dam workers brought their families with them when they relocated to Oregon to work on the project. Moreover, unlike at Contractor's General, Mason City Hospital's doctors not only took care of injured and sick Kaiser employees; they also cared for their women and children, too.

The workers demanded a health-care plan that covered dependents, and Kaiser complied, paying a little more to Garfield for each employee with a family.

The health-care and the construction enterprises quickly became interdependent. Kaiser wanted healthy employees and provided Garfield with a prospective, per capita fee to do so—which we now know as *capitation*. Garfield taught Kaiser about the advantages of prevention and safety over crisis-oriented medical care, and Kaiser taught Garfield about industrially derived efficiencies that allowed his relatively small staff to handle over 40,000 treatments a year.

The arrangement was so mutually beneficial that Garfield went on to work with Kaiser in Richmond, California, and Portland, Oregon, where the company had shipyards that built the so-called Liberty Ships, which were mass-produced cargo vessels made in large numbers during World War II. The ships originally took over 200 days to finish, but with practice and the war imperative, the average build-time eventually dropped to 42 days. Liberty Ships were produced in 13 states by 15 companies in 18 shipyards. Prefabricated sections were shipped on railroad cars from around the country to the ports where they were assembled, much as the pieces of Eli Whitney's musket had been in an earlier generation. The fabrication methods were modeled after the ones Ford Motor used for cars before the war. Inevitably, the shipyards began to compete, and a formal competition to assemble one of these mass-produced vessels began at 12:01 AM, November 8, 1942.

A completed Liberty Ship was 440 feet long and 55 feet wide and had two steam-powered boilers and 250,000 parts; it weighed 14 million pounds. In a remarkable achievement, even by today's standards, the SS *Robert E. Peary* was completed in just 4 days, 15 hours and 29 minutes from the time its keel was laid. The winning shipyard was the Permanente Metals Corporation (a Kaiser Company) Number 2 Yard in Richmond, California.

Kaiser Construction was successful in building ships, roads, aqueducts and dams quickly and efficiently because it changed, adapted and adopted new techniques. Welding replaced riveting, allowing faster and lighter joins. Women were hired into the workforce to replace the men who had joined the army, and Rosie the Riveter became Wendy the Welder.

At the conclusion of the Grand Coulee project, like most young men of his age, Garfield had already been drafted to enter active duty in the army when Kaiser approached him about setting up a health-care plan for the

Richmond shipyards. Already in uniform and about to head to India, the ever-willing physician offered to help get a plan off the ground before he left. But Kaiser had bigger ideas. He sent his lieutenant, the fixer, Alonzo Ordway, to Washington. Ordway met with Franklin D. Roosevelt and persuaded him that Garfield and his medical model were essential to the Kaiser Company's critical shipbuilding enterprise. Roosevelt released him from his service obligation so that he could start a health plan for the steelworkers.

Garfield quickly purchased a four-story, unused building in Oakland that was once an obstetric facility, refurbished it and painted it pink—Henry Kaiser's favorite color. Within months the doctor had incorporated the Permanente Foundation Hospital, Permanente Health Plan and Sidney R. Garfield physician group—all during the summer of 1942. By 1944, Garfield was running four hospitals with 790 beds, and the health plan was caring for 200,000 patients.

Like the previous enterprises, the Permanente Health Plan was restricted to the employees and families of the Kaiser companies. As such, its physicians were largely sheltered from the attentions of medicine-at-large, which didn't see the arrangement as a significant threat to the fee-for-service payment scheme that the American Medical Association (AMA) believed in. But things changed with the end of the war.

By the middle of 1945, the shipbuilding efforts had wound down, and tens of thousands of workers had moved on to civilian jobs in other parts of the country. The Kaiser health enterprise would have shrunk as rapidly as its war-related business did were it not for the fact that Kaiser Permanente decided to open its doors to the public at a time when, according to *Forbes Magazine,* 90 percent of the general public could not afford traditional fee-for-service medical care. Membership in the Kaiser plan soared immediately, setting the grounds for what would quickly become a war on Kaiser doctors by the rest of organized medicine. Organized medicine's food source, its patients, was at stake.

Professional medical societies labeled the Kaiser Permanente model "corporate" and "socialized" medicine—the latter equivalent to saying it was Communist. Its physicians were described as unethical and were denied membership in local and national professional societies. They were therefore unable to take board examinations or be privileged to admit patients to non-Kaiser hospitals. They were shunned by the medical community. Garfield's medical license was even suspended briefly.

The rest of the medical world viewed the Kaiser model as a threat, and not merely in a competitive sense. There was a fear, not unwarranted as it turned out, that Garfield's model might spread like a virulent, communicable virus and contaminate the rest of medicine. The Kaiser model looked like a typical government-run plan to the American Medical Association, whose doctors were perfectly happy with the fee-for-service approach. The latter were vehemently against governmental health care. And the two approaches couldn't be more different.

The key to Garfield's success was the fact that he was prepaid, or "*imbursed*" with a "per-patient" sum of money. In other words, his physicians were given a yearly budget to work with to cover all patients enrolled in the plan, which amounted to the per-capita rate times the number of insured heads (*caput* is the Latin word for head). In the fee-for-service world, on the other hand, physicians were *re*imbursed, *after* the fact, for whatever care was provided to the patient; there was *no* budget. And while one would like to believe that the care provided by doctors under these differing models would have no impact on the ultimate outcomes for patients, the incentives were certainly radically different.

The folks who ran the Kaiser plan, like the ones who ran the Kaiser companies, cared about efficiency and looked for ways to increase productivity and reduce cost. The Kaiser Health Plan had its roots in the recognition that a healthier workforce was a more productive one, and its workers were encouraged to stay healthy, as is evident in this World War II–era exhortation from Kaiser management to its workforce: "Unless preventative measures are taken, a total of 720,000 working days a year [at the Richmond Shipyards] will be lost due to accidents occurring away from work and due to illness. With those lost days, you could build ten ships. With those lost days you could earn more than four million dollars. Such waste is tragic when the Nation is fighting for its very life."[3]

The Kaiser plan followed industrial precepts using standardized assembly lines focused on quick turnover so that patients were registered, evaluated by the nurse, seen by the doctor and out the door holding a newly filled prescription with clockwork efficiency. Its managers attempted to improve productivity and reduce turnover and absenteeism through comprehensive health management, including nutrition and child care for offspring and prepared meals for female workers who constituted a significant percentage of the workforce during the war. A cartoon from the era shows a "distraught and angry woman with a burning pot in the background, holding a pan to heat a baby bottle in one hand while thrusting the telephone receiver at her screaming child with the other. The caption read[s] 'Here [to the infant], you talk to the foreman. Explain why I didn't show up for work today.'"[4]

The company also took on a more intrusive role by monitoring the use of first-aid stations and medical facilities in an attempt to identify potential malingerers. Unlike his more patriarchal counterpart in the traditional doctor-patient relationship, the Kaiser physician was described a "*facilitator* in the maintenance of health." Henry Kaiser himself described the Permanente outpatient clinic, which was designed to keep his workers productive, as "an assembly line of men."[5]

While the traditional medical world, as embodied by the American Medical Association, abhorred the Kaiser mass-production medical philosophy and scorned its doctors as cogs in a machine, Kaiser clinicians actually pioneered advances in preventative and occupational medicine. Eventually the battle between the Kaiser model and the AMA played out on a national stage in Congress as Kaiser pushed for a national health plan built around the prepayment model, and societies such as the AMA and the American Hospital Association pushed back. Democrats tended to align with the former, while Republicans supported the latter.

In a very real sense, the divide between the two worlds came to be aligned along the socioeconomic plane between blue-collar workers and their acute diseases, such as syphilis and tuberculosis, and the more chronic diseases of the affluent, which were studied at highbrow academic institutions such as Stanford and the University of California, San Francisco (UCSF). The latter produced specialists certified by boards of examiners; those very boards and also the regional medical societies refused, for many years, to certify or even acknowledge Kaiser physicians, who were predominantly general practitioners.

In retrospect, both combatants can legitimately claim a Pyrrhic victory. In the 1940s, over 75 percent of practicing physicians described themselves as general practitioners, while 20 years later more than half were specialists. Only 30 percent of today's doctors are what are now called *primary care providers.* So the specialists won, although we now bemoan the absence of enough frontline practitioners. On the other hand, the fee-for-service model so cherished by the AMA in the 1950s and 1960s is slowly dying today. A significant proportion of medical care now is prepaid and has been strongly influenced by the Kaiser health-maintenance philosophy.

The medical world we know today is a hybrid. We have a highly special-ized, evolutionarily diversified population of physicians, from internists and surgeons to cardiologists and urologists to interventional radiologists, pedi-atric neonatologists and echocardiologists. These specialists, sub-specialists and sub-sub-specialists are analogous to the skilled artisans of yore—the weavers, glassblowers or silversmiths—and emanate from the same appren-ticeship tradition. We also have a newly evolving class of medical specialists whose roots spring from the Kaiser assembly-line approach to health care and maintenance. These are the hospitalists and nocturnalists whose job is to facilitate and streamline the flow of patients through the health system, just as the welders and painters did in the Oakland shipyards.

Welding was one of the advances that allowed American shipyards to ramp up from a production of 23 ships in the 1930s to 10,000 in the 1940s, which was an average of a ship a day from the San Francisco Bay Area alone. The welders' work was made easier by pre-positioning the parts so that the welder could work with her hands down, below the waist. Vertical elements, such as walls, were turned horizontal for welding, and ceilings were inverted. The piece was brought to the worker rather than the worker traveling to the piece.

The same drive for increased efficiency spurred the evolution of the hospitalist, who stays in the hospital where his "work"—hospitalized patients—comes to him. *Nocturnalists*, like Sarah Stone, Raj Desai and Frank Delacourt, whom I introduced at the beginning of this chapter, are essentially medical shift workers. Similarly, overtaxed obstetricians are diminishing in number due to a variety of lifestyle and malpractice issues and no longer want to be on call every night for the delivery of every one of their patients, as they once were. A new specialty field, the obstetric *laborist*, who takes calls for deliveries only, has evolved to fill this niche—and to take another spot along the assembly line. The *admitologist* sits between the office-based practitioner or emergency room and the hospitalist, assess-ing and pre-positioning newly admitted patients, doing the paperwork and writing the orders.

Medical efficiency experts now use explicit analogies to an industrial model of health care, and they adopt streamlining approaches from the computer industry. Computers use parallel processing to increase speed, much as the hospitalist can proceed about her business while, in parallel, the admitologist preprocesses new patients for her.

The relationship between Sidney Garfield and Henry Kaiser, which began on a business footing as a way for Kaiser to keep his workers happy and productive, evolved dramatically over the rest of their lives. Kaiser's first wife, Bess, to whom he was married for 43 years, developed nephritis, an inflammation of the kidneys, in 1950. Henry did not want her to die in a hospital, so Garfield set up a field hospital in their apartment and deputized his head nurse, Alyce Chester, to move in and care for the dying woman over the last six months of her life.

Bess died in March 1951. Less than a month later, and despite the protests of his children and colleagues, the newly widowed 68-year-old Kaiser announced that he and Alyce—who was 34, the mother of a young son and an attractive, dynamic woman—would marry.

After her marriage to Kaiser, nurse Alyce "Ale" Kaiser remained in a lead administrative role with Garfield, who was running the Kaiser Permanente medical empire, including its medical facilities and physician group. He was also planning the development of new hospitals in the Bay area.

Perhaps not coincidentally, Henry's interests in and meddling with the medical side of his business increased dramatically now that he was married to one of its principals. The new Kaiser couple's micromanagement didn't stop with patient care. They decided to cure Garfield of his bachelorhood.

Within a year, Ale's younger, married sister, Helen Peterson, also a pretty woman, divorced her current husband, making her eligible as a match for the handsome, successful and single Garfield. Ale and Henry, Helen and Sidney and a few close friends jumped on Kaiser's private DC-3 and flew from San Francisco to Reno late one night, on very short notice for a city hall wedding ceremony. As a friend who attended the wedding described it: "Dr. Garfield was living with us when we got the call. Mrs. Cutting and I, and the Neighbors had been salmon fishing that day. We got home wet and tired and dirty, just getting to bed, when the phone rang. 'Mr. Kaiser wants you down at the airport right away. Sid's getting married.' Sid then got on the phone and said would we bring his suit and a clean shirt to the airport. We flew to Reno and Sid got married, and (then we) flew back."[6]

Shortly thereafter, the Garfields moved in next door to the Kaiser mansion outside of Oakland. Kaiser and his onetime protégé were now neighbors and brothers-in-law. A friend described nightly cocktail hours between the two couples, at which there were "the most horrendous fights, embarrassing arguments and explosions" between the two men, which Garfield invariably lost.[7] The couples remained close until the end of Kaiser's life in 1967, at the age of 85 on the island of Hawaii, where he had retired.

Kaiser and Garfield were both visionaries, albeit of a different stripe. Kaiser was one of America's great industrialists and self-made men, in the mold of Henry Ford and Bill Gates. He is quoted as having said: "I make progress by having people around me who are smarter than I am and listening to them. And I assume everyone is smarter about something than I am." He also said: "You can't sit on the lid of progress. If you do, you will be blown to pieces."[8]

Garfield was equally ambitious and far thinking. He pioneered and championed the concept of wellness, in which there was a compact between the physician and the patient by which both would work to maintain the good health of the latter. "Personally," he said, "I am more interested in the future than the past."[9]

Late in his career, Garfield published a signature and startlingly prescient 1970 article in *Scientific American* entitled "The Delivery of Medical Care."[10] In it, he envisioned a medical future in which computers would maintain records and help to triage patients into one of three categories: the "worried well," who needed education rather than expensive care; patients with legitimate chronic conditions who would receive "preventative maintenance;" and the "truly ill," who would be managed by group practice physicians providing acute and intensive care.

Garfield believed that the cure to the failures of traditional, fee-for-service, crisis-management medicine was a new health-and-wellness-oriented system, enhanced by computer algorithms and electronic medical records. This system, he believed, would hold "great promise for the provision of truly preventative care. We need no longer generalize, but instead we can instruct each individual about what he should do for optimal health on the basis of his own, updated profile."[11]

CHAPTER 9

FOR ONE GOOD NEW SUIT OF CLOTHES

Hi Dr. Smith,

Thank you so much for letting me figure out how to schedule my in vitro fertilization *during my rotation in the ICU. Right now, I'm supposed to do the egg harvest around mid-month and then the implantation two days later. If it works out that way, I am supposed to be on call the day of harvest and I think I'll need to take that day off, since it is done under sedation, and then I have to be on two days of bed rest after the implantation. You're the best, S.*

A friend of mine who directs an ICU training program at another institution received an email very much like this one not too long ago and forwarded it to get my reaction. It was from a resident who was slated to begin a week or two later one of the toughest rotations during her residency—a month in the intensive care unit caring for the sickest patients in the hospital. This email, with its inherent assumptions, serves as a perfect illustration of the degree to which medical training has changed over the last few decades and a glimpse of what the practice of medicine will look like in the future.

Put bluntly, people didn't get pregnant during their residency 25 years ago. Sure, they engaged in all of the preliminaries—sometimes even during work hours—but I can't think of a single resident in a direct-care discipline (as opposed to radiology or pathology, for example) who interrupted her training for a pregnancy, planned or otherwise, while I was a resident. It just wasn't done. Families, food and sleep were all secondary to training.

The ICU rotation has always been one of the heaviest months, during which residents are continuously engaged in round-the-clock care of the sickest of the sick. As an indicator of how dramatically things have changed, not only was the resident who wrote that email actually hoping, almost planning, to become pregnant during her residency, she had actually scheduled her elective infertility treatment concurrent with what might arguably be her *toughest residency month*. To cap it off, she knew she'd need to take several days off during that month for bed rest of one sort or another, and she only let my colleague in on that secret a week before her rotation was to begin, well after the schedule had already been written. And in one final perverse wrinkle, she later told my colleague that she was actually planning on going into critical care as a career choice.

As I thought about the email, several competing thoughts ran through my mind. Very prominent was a sense of admiration for the resident: this was a masterstroke of multitasking on the one hand and, in a sense, brilliantly manipulative on the other. A couple that needs to resort to in vitro fertilization (IVF) in order to conceive a child has obviously failed with more traditional measures, and the treatment is not always successful the first time. Some couples go through several rounds of IVF and even then are never successful even with this very medically sophisticated method of making a baby.

The so-called live birth rate for a course of IVF in a 30-something female is around 33 percent. This resident knew that there was a good likelihood that she'd need to go through several attempts before conceiving. She also knew that if she took a month off for each course, she'd need to pay those months back at the end of her residency; and, of course, if she was successful, she'd need to interrupt her training for the delivery of the baby, time that would also be tacked on.

So she had made the calculation that, to the extent possible, she would conduct her medical training and family development activities concurrently, which is a course of action that, as I mentioned, would have been inconceivable, so to say, to a female medical resident a few short years ago. A cautionary note that ran through my mind was the fact that the sleeplessness and the stresses of the ICU rotation were unlikely to have a positive impact on the outcome of the IVF attempt.

The thing that was strikingly absent from my initial reaction, and that of my colleague, was a sense of outrage that this mere trainee had the audacity to attempt to dictate the terms of her indenture in this fashion. Back in my day, not only would a communiqué of this sort (no email then) have been shocking, it would have been a career ender. But there's been a major shift in the balance of power between residents and their physician educators since those days. Until relatively recently, the resident was a kind of a serf—admittedly a serf with high hopes—but still essentially a human beast of burden. Now, the resident is more of a squire: a young lordling with more rights and fewer responsibilities than in times of yore.

In order to best understand the difference between the old days and now, it is necessary to go back to the night of March 4, 1984, to a hospital then known as New York Hospital, where an 18-year-old college freshman was admitted with a fever, chills and agitation. The woman had recently undergone a tooth extraction and then developed a low-grade fever. Despite beginning antibiotic therapy, her symptoms got worse instead of better.

Her temperature increased to 103 degrees Fahrenheit, and there were too many white blood cells in her bloodstream, often indicative of bacterial infection. She had a history of depression and was taking an antidepressant. The doctors who admitted her weren't sure what to call her problem but cautiously decided to bring her in for observation and hydration.

Doctors typically use what's called a *differential diagnosis* to categorize the list of likely possibilities for a given set of findings. The usual goal is to go about a series of tests to cross things *off* of the differential, thereby homing in on an answer. The differential for a high temperature, white count and agitation is pretty big, however, and includes a whole range of infections and drug reactions.

After a stay in the emergency room, the patient was sent to a hospital floor bed. She would have been one of several admissions, or what are known in residency vernacular as "hits," for Dr. Luise Weinstein, the admitting intern that night. Weinstein, only eight months out of medical school, was also caring for 40 other patients scattered elsewhere in the hospital. She was supervised by a more senior resident, Dr. Gregg Stone, who was only a year further along in his training.

As was typical, Weinstein and Stone both evaluated the patient and arrived at a plan. Like the admitting doctors, they weren't exactly sure what was going on and tentatively labeled the problem a "viral syndrome with hysterical symptoms." One of the interventions they prescribed was a small dose of meperidine, brand-named Demerol, which is a narcotic sometimes used to treat shaking in patients with shivering during chemotherapy or after anesthesia.

The two young doctors ran their proposed diagnosis and course of action by a senior clinician over the phone, in this case the family's physician, who approved it. The patient's parents stayed with her at the hospital until about 3 AM on March 5, and then went home. Stone, the second-year resident, then headed off to catch a little sleep in a building across the street from the hospital.

Unlike Stone, however, Weinstein wasn't expected to sleep that night. Her job was to act as the first responder. While Stone would see all of the new patients with her, she would see the admissions first and handle all phone calls from the nighttime floor staff about patient problems, putting out all of the little fires along the way: the temperature spikes, the urinary retentions, the fecal impactions and so on. She'd call Stone if anything got complicated or beyond her, but a good intern was known as a "wall," and a good wall stopped all but the most grievous of breaches from getting through to the second-year resident. Calling for help was "weak."

In that era, every house officer was expected to act like a soldier and to defend his position. Absenteeism for whatever reason that didn't involve traction or incarceration was unconscionably weak, because it meant that some other house officer had to fill in. Pregnancy not involving traction or incarceration, and the consequent prolonged absence from duty, would have been fatally weak and wasn't to be imagined.

Weinstein got several calls that night about her "hysterical" patient, whose body temperature had risen alarmingly and who had begun to thrash around the bed. She prescribed a restraining vest, called a Posey, that was tied to the bed with a belt, and soft extremity "cuffs" intended to keep the patient from falling out of bed or pulling out medical catheters. Weinstein complemented the belts with pharmacologic suspenders in the form of a sedative called *haloperidol*, typically used to treat psychosis.

Tied up with her other patients, the young doctor never got back to see her charge before the woman's temperature reached 107 degrees at 6:30 AM on the first morning of her admission, a few hours after her parents had left her bedside. Weinstein ordered cold compresses and a cooling blanket, but shortly thereafter, the patient had a cardiac arrest—her heart stopped. Despite intensive cardiopulmonary resuscitation for an hour, the young woman was unable to be revived because the heart and brain no longer function properly when the body is that hot. She died. And it was as a result of her death that medical training changed irreversibly from what had traditionally been an apprenticeship, in which the trainee was expected to extend herself almost infinitely to fill the available workload, to something much more sensible.

The young patient's name was Libby Zion, and while we still don't know exactly what caused her death, the general consensus is that she developed a very unusual, very bad, drug interaction between an antidepressant she was taking before admission and the small dose of Demerol prescribed by Weinstein. To be fair, Zion arrived at the hospital with a fever and was agitated in the emergency room before she received any Demerol (that's why she was admitted in the first place) and she was taking other prescription medications. Today's papers are full of stories of young people who die from complications involving combinations of licit and illicit drugs, but this case changed medicine permanently because Libby Zion had a powerful advocate.

Libby's father, Sydney Zion, was a larger-than-life lawyer, journalist and man-about-town in New York City. A columnist for the *New York Daily News* at the time of her death, he also wrote at various times for the *New York Times, New York Magazine* and the *New York Post*. Zion smoked big cigars, talked loudly, wore a fedora and held court at prominent city watering holes, including the Yale Club. He had gone to Yale Law School after finishing his undergraduate years at the University of Pennsylvania. Zion was also friendly with many of the powerful players in the city, and he didn't buy the hospital's explanation for his daughter's death, which was that she had died of some unusual infection. Like any parent, he wanted to know *why* his child had died, and among his many skills, he was a very good investigative journalist.

Zion investigated. The more he learned, the more he sensed that the hospital's "unusual infection" explanation didn't make sense and that her death was much more likely due to what we now call an *adverse drug reaction* between two drugs that act together to cause a surge in the levels of

a brain chemical called *serotonin.* Serotonin syndrome has many mani-
festations, including sweating, twitching, hyperactive reflexes, agitation,
increased heart rate and blood pressure and, most prominently, high fever.
Unrecognized and untreated, the syndrome can progress rapidly to muscle
breakdown, kidney failure, seizures and death.

Zion also didn't understand why they used restraints and medications
to control his increasingly agitated daughter that night. As he put it: "They
gave her a drug that was destined to kill her, then ignored her except to tie
her down like a dog."[1] Parenthetically, and due in some part to this case,
hospital regulatory agencies carefully scrutinize the use of restraints today,
and their use is much less common than it was in the 1980s.

Zion came to refer to the death of his daughter as a "murder," laying a
large part of the blame on the hospital and its staffing pattern. He wrote an
op-ed column in which he stated: "You don't need kindergarten to know
that a resident working a 36-hour shift is in no condition to make any kind
of judgment call—let alone life and death."[2] Zion loudly vented his opin-
ions about the hospital and traditional medical education being complicit
in Libby's death. He told anyone who would listen, and he had many friends
among those in journalism and in power. Largely due to his efforts, the
image of the medical trainee underwent a startling change.

The young Drs. Kildare and Casey of the 1940s, 1950s and 1960s were
attractive, noble and tireless round-the-clock advocates for patients during
their years as medical trainees, and the poster children exemplified the breed
for the vast majority of the public through the early 1980s. But by 1990, and
largely as a result of the efforts of Sydney Zion, a new picture of the medical house officer began to creep into publications like the *New York Times,*
the *Washington Post* and *Newsweek,* as well as television productions like *60
Minutes.* The interns and residents described in these media were exhausted,
disheveled and forgetful. At best, they looked barely capable of managing
their own lives, much less the lives of 30 to 40 sick, hospitalized patients.

Two years after Libby's death, the Manhattan district attorney, Robert
Morgenthau, concluded that the issues surrounding Libby Zion's death were
sufficiently problematic that he allowed a grand jury to consider murder
charges against the doctors who cared for her. While the grand jury ultimately concluded that there was no basis for a criminal prosecution, it issued
a report strongly criticizing "the supervision of interns and house officers at
a hospital in New York County."[3]

In response, the state's commissioner of health, David Axelrod, convened the Ad Hoc Advisory Committee on Emergency Services to evaluate the training and supervision of medical house officers in New York. Axelrod asked Bertrand Bell, a primary care physician from the Albert Einstein College of Medicine, to head the commission. His selection of Bell as chairman was a strong signal as to the direction the "evaluation" was intended to take. Bell was a long-time critic of the lack of supervision of house staff in New York hospitals.

The term *house staff* dates back to an era when residents were "on call" around the clock, dating back to the period between the 1910 Flexner Report and World War II. These young doctors were typically unmarried young men from an upper-middle-class background who elected to do specialized training in hospital medicine. In the beginning, hospital medicine was a specialized track; most doctors completed their apprenticeship and went directly into general practice without a period of residency in a hospital.

The young doctors who elected to become hospital residents or house staff essentially moved into the hospital for a stretch of their lives, to be immediately available whenever needed. But given the realities of that time, and what one could actually do when called, they weren't really *needed* that much. Unlike today's throbbing 24-hour-a-day enterprises, the hospitals of that era didn't have laboratories or medical devices. There weren't emergency wards through which patients like Libby Zion could be admitted around-the-clock. Helicopters didn't fly in with new patients from far away. In fact, there were no helicopters, beepers, or overhead public address systems in hospitals. If a nurse needed a doctor, she went and found him in his quarters and timidly asked him to come see the patient. And it would have had to have been a pretty serious issue to rouse a sleeping doctor back then.

By the time Libby Zion was admitted in the wee hours of Monday, March 5, 1984, house officers at busy hospitals rarely slept. Their beepers went off constantly, and interns walked around in white coats soiled with dirt or bodily fluids. They carried packs of index cards on which they recorded each patient's history and lab data, often illegibly. Their pockets sagged with quick guides to antibiotics along with medical instruments and comfort food. They didn't always smell good or have clean hair. These were the best and the brightest of their generation: the young people of the era who had "gotten into medical school" at a time when there was fierce competition for every spot.

The gentleman "houseman" of the turn of the century had morphed—through a slow but inexorable process of mission creep—to the 1980s-era, sleepwalking, error-prone automaton that Sydney Zion believed was responsible for the "murder" of his daughter. To be fair, neither Gregg Stone nor Luise Weinstein, the house officers who cared for her, believed that fatigue played any role in Libby's death, even years later.

But none would question the fact that her parents' rage—perhaps misplaced—against the environment in which she died changed the rules of medical training forever. Prior to then, residency was a form of extended boot camp analogous to Hell Week of the Navy SEALs—except that it went on for years—and, as with the SEALs, its survivors believed they were the stronger for the experience. But the recommendations that ultimately came from the Ad Hoc Advisory Commission on Emergency Services, which came to be known as the Bell Commission, suggested limits to what had previously been a limitless resource.

The Bell commission produced a set of guidelines including stipulations that residents could not work more than 80 hours in a week or 24 consecutive hours. Before, it was not uncommon for residents to start work in the hospital on the morning of one day and not leave—and often not sleep—until the afternoon of the next. That call pattern might repeat on an every-third- or even an every-other-night basis, so it was possible for residents to get only one good night's sleep, every two nights, for years on end. In some particularly harsh cases, a resident could start work on a Friday morning and not leave the hospital until the following Monday afternoon—a *continuous* stretch of more than 80 hours. This was the way I, and most of my contemporaries, spent our residencies.

One would intuitively think that the impetus for change should have come from within the medical profession rather than from an external, governmentally appointed body. But there had been surprisingly little protest from residents across the Western world, even as the workload increased and the length of residencies stretched, in some cases, to a full decade—ten years of low pay, sleep deprivation and delayed gratification.

Interns went on strike in the United Kingdom for a brief period in the 1970s, and there was periodic talk around the world of unionization. But there was never any substantive organized push-back about the increasingly intolerable work conditions. Once done, in fact, a newly minted surgeon might actually brag that he had spent a "decade with Dick" (the tough-as-nails former chairman of one prominent department of surgery). A lawyer or banker graduating from the same college class would have had a ten-year head start in the creation of family and net worth on a roommate who had gone into medicine.

There was also no push for change from senior physicians during that era. They had survived medical boot camp themselves and were the ultimate beneficiaries of the cheap and seemingly inexhaustible resource represented by the resident workforce. In effect, they were often able to sleep at night as their apprentices toiled. In fact, many senior doctors bridled at the Bell commission's recommendations, protesting that one could not become a qualified physician without having continuously cared for patients through the first critical hours of their illnesses.

They argued that the multiple hand-offs necessitated by work-hour restrictions would result in lost information and a loss in the continuity of care of individual patients. One frequently adopted solution to these restrictions was the institution of a "night-float" system, wherein designated residents arrived late in the afternoon to relieve the day-resident for that night. The night-float resident might do a week or a month of nights covering a team of patients for the nocturnal 12-hour stretch; this necessitated a hand-off of care from one individual to another every half-day.

Despite protests from the medical community, New York State adopted the recommendations of the Bell commission in 1989. While not all institutions initially adhered to these recommendations, by 2003 the national Accreditation Council for Graduate Medical Education, the ACGME, made reduced work hours mandatory for accreditation of any residency in any medical discipline anywhere in the United States. Thereafter, if a residency violated the work-hour restrictions, it lost accreditation—and no accreditation meant no residents. Similar regulations are now in place in most of Europe, Australia, New Zealand, Canada and the United Kingdom. In fact, some European countries now limit the maximum allowable weekly duty hours to as few as 48.

In effect, the ACGME threatened that if a residency mistreated its trainees, it would lose its official recognition, and the hospital would thereby lose its cheap, semi-skilled workforce. While various attempts to unionize medical trainees had failed over previous years, the work-hour rules stuck. As a result, the balance of power between the resident and the training program began to change. Because residents could now anonymously report work-hour violations on the part of their employer programs, they suddenly

acquired power. In fact, the following news item shows just how much leverage residents gained with the national implementation of the Bell commission recommendations by the ACGME:

> Yale-New Haven Medical Center's surgical resident program
> recently failed to meet ACGME standards and could lose its
> accreditation as of June 30, 2003.... News reports said the 50-
> resident program was cited for work-hour violations, deficient
> supervision of residents... [and that] residents worked more than
> 100 hours a week and failed to follow ACGME rules limiting
> on-call duty to no more than one day out of three and requiring
> one day off every seven.... [The] chief of staff at the hospital was
> quoted as saying the program would spend $1 million to bring it
> back up to standards [by] hiring up to a dozen physicians' assis-
> tants and nurse practitioners and bringing other physicians and
> residents in.[4]

With the citation of this prominent academic surgical program, the
ACGME fired a warning shot across the bow of every one of the thousands
of medical training programs in the country, showing how serious it was
about duty-hour violations. And with the announcement that it was willing to spend a seven-figure sum to rectify the problem, Yale-New Haven
Medical Center indicated how seriously it took the threat.

Absent residents, surgery at the medical center would have slowed dramatically, costing the center many more millions than it was willing to spend
on the solution. Of equal importance was the potential negative impact on
the surgery program's prestige: If it were to lose certification for even a brief
period, the best applicants would no longer look at Yale's program for fear
that they might not become board-certified in surgery at the end of years of
training.

One contemporaneous medical student blog posting said: "The recently
appointed [Yale surgery] chairman... seems caught with his pants down.
The place seems to be in a shambles, and I feel bad for any students who
matched there this year. My advice would be to take one of the hundreds of
open [spots elsewhere]...."[5]

When all was said and done, with the institution of the duty-hour limitations resulting from the tragic events surrounding Libby Zion's death,

there was suddenly a new world order in medical training. The old ways, the ways of the medical apprentice, were no longer the good ways.

The ACGME was originally designed to make sure that residencies were meeting educational requirements for specific training programs, for example, that a surgery resident did at least a certain number of proctored gall bladder operations before being certified. With the institution of duty-hour limits, however, the ACGME became a sort of institutional social worker— one who could remove the "children" from their home-away-from-home if they weren't being treated properly—and the children got the message.

The men and women who choose to enter a medical career are smart and hard-working and clearly able to take the long view. In many specialty areas, they delay economic gratification for well over a decade after graduating from medical school. These smart young people immediately recognized the implications of the showdown between the ACGME and the Yale-New Haven Hospital. They understood from that time forward that, merely by sending a complaint to the ACGME about duty hours or working conditions in their residency, they had the power to bring the program to its knees. So, what was formerly a private arrangement between training program and trainee was now subject to outside scrutiny and intervention. The Bell commission had been officially tasked with setting reasonable boundaries around the amount of time that New York medical residents could be expected to function effectively in the delivery of medical care, but their unspoken, and perhaps unrecognized, mission was to change a method of training that dated back to the Middle Ages—the apprenticeship.

Craft guilds emerged in the chaotic medieval period to ensure the protection and mutual aid of individuals in the same occupation. Their charters included rules prohibiting illicit trading by members, provisions for the sick and disabled craftsmen and provisions for the protection of the craftsmen or -women (there were women's guilds for weavers, for example) as they plied their trades. There were guilds for masons, carpenters, painters, candle makers, cobblers and apothecaries, among others, and the benefits of the guild structure included rigid control over the business model. Guilds were monopolistic; prices for goods were fixed, and there were also high standards of quality. The guilds maintained tight control over the amount of "product" by restricting membership to a select cadre of highly trained, carefully selected master craftsmen.

Much as today's path to becoming a physician begins more than a decade earlier, medieval parents would apprentice their child to a master when the boy was between ten and fifteen years of age. The apprentice would board with the master for a period of five to ten years while he learned the fundamentals of his trade.

The apprentice got up in the morning, gathered the wood and started the metalworker's fire or sharpened the carpenter's planes and saws. Then, perhaps, he would eat breakfast at the master's table. The apprentice worked hard all day, and he lived and breathed his trade. He wasn't paid; in fact his parents typically paid a fee for room and board, and he wasn't allowed to marry. If he was successful, an apprentice might go on to become a journeyman, the next level up in the tiered system. As part of the terms of his contract, or indenture, the apprentice would be issued a set of tools at the conclusion of his training by the master and could hire himself out to practice his trade as a journeyman.

Unlike the apprentice, a journeyman was paid for his work and emancipated from his master. In fact, an unambitious journeyman could remain at that level forever by living off his wages as an assistant. In order to finally become a master, the journeyman had to complete a "master piece" acceptable to the guild he wished to enter. For example, a journeyman watchmaker might make an innovative or beautifully crafted watch, while a joiner might make an ornate cabinet. The guild's acceptance of the master piece meant that the new master could open his own workshop, hire an apprentice workforce—and marry.

The apprentice-journeyman-master model survives today in many formats. We still have, for example, master plumbers and electricians in the skilled trades. Apprenticeships are common through a wide variety of fields in Europe and Asia. And the professions, which have historically been distinguished from the trades by virtue of a more formal education in a university setting, have the three-tiered progression from bachelor's to master's and, finally, doctoral degrees. Medicine was one of the three original professions, the others being law and divinity, but medical training has historically combined elements of both apprenticeship and professional training.

Luise Weinstein and Gregg Stone, like every medical resident, had already graduated into the medical profession by the time they started their internship; they had their medical degree. But then, and only then, did they begin the real, practical part of medical training—as indentured, apprentice physicians. The typical indenture of an eighteenth-century apprentice contained language like the following from the contract between James Franklin and his uncle Benjamin:

> Witnessth, That James Franklin late of Newport in Rhode island, And now of Philadelphia in Pennsylvania Hath put himself...Apprentice to Benjamin Franklin of the City of Philadelphia, Printer to learn his Art, Trade, and Mystery, and...to serve the said Benjamin Franklin from the Day of the Date herof, for...Seven Years...During all which Term, the said Apprentice his said Master faithfully shall serve, his Secrets keep, his lawfull Commands everywhere readily obey.
>
> He shall not commit Fornication, nor contract Matrimony within the said Term. At Cards, Dice, or any other unlawful Game, he shall not play....He shall not absent himself Day nor Night from his said Master's Service, without his Leave: Nor haunt Ale-houses, Taverns, or Play-houses.
>
> And the said Master shall use the utmost of his Endeavour to teach or cause to be taught or instructed the said Apprentice in the Trade or Mystery of Printing and procure and provide for him sufficient Meat, Drink, Cloaths, Lodging and Washing fitting to an Apprentice, during the said Term of Seven Years and at the Expiration thereof shall give him one good new Suit of Cloaths, besides his common Apparel.[6]

Like James Franklin, the typical Revolutionary War–era apprentice contracted to a multi-year relationship with his master, during which time he would faithfully serve, keep his secrets, obey his commands, avoid activities that might result in an inconvenient offspring, stay out of casinos and bars and, above all, promise to be available day and night. The pre-Bell commission-era medical resident signed on for a pretty similar deal: years of uncomplaining servitude without time for fun and games, in return for which she received meal vouchers, a call-room bed, a beeper, a pocketbook full of medical secrets and "one good new" white coat. The balance of power in both relationships rested totally with the educator. But the work-hour rules put forth by the Bell commission, and subsequently adopted nationally by the ACGME, eventually changed the relationship between the student physician and the educator in ways that have already begun to change the practice of medicine irrevocably.

The relationship between the apprentice and the master directly mirrored the one between a parent and a child; in fact, the apprentice's parent typically cosigned the indenture and effectively transferred parental responsibilities to the master by so doing. Once the apprentice became a member of the master's household, he didn't break the rules, gripe about the food or question his work hours. Sure, he might write home to his real parents about hazing from older apprentices in the shop or, worse, about the beatings he received at the hands of his master. But the only way to advance in the field was by persevering for the term of the contract.

As medical residents in the 1980s, we had the same deal: put up with the deprivations of sleep, autonomy and salary during residency with the expectation of a stable, rewarding, lifelong professional career at the end of the tunnel. Everyone—the medical students, the residents, the master doctors and the public—"got it": doctors put up with grueling residencies in exchange for a lucrative, stable career. The Libby Zion case and the resulting Bell commission changed all that by introducing a third party into the equation in the form of organizations, like the ACGME, that began to observe and regulate the work conditions of medical trainees.

The work-hour limitations recommended by the Bell commission and adopted by New York State are now the standard. While there have been a few studies of resident fatigue and medical errors, it's hard to be certain whether there has been a net benefit to patient safety. It is becoming clear, however, that the Bell commission's report has already resulted in effects on medical training and practice as profound of those of the Flexner Report almost a century earlier. In fact, the 2008 recommendations from the United States Institute of Medicine further limit a continuous stretch of duty to 16 hours (down from 24) and suggest 5-hour naps between 10 PM and 8 AM.[7]

The organizational and legislative bodies that arrived at these limits invariably struggled to balance three objectives: improved resident well-being, enhanced patient safety and the establishment of appropriate educational opportunities for the trainees. There are huge financial and workforce implications to their conclusions. For example, in order to comply with one version of work-hour rules, researchers estimated that 8,000 to 10,000 additional advanced health-care providers would need to be added to the health-care rolls.

There are now two almost equally sized groups of physicians in the workforce: an older cadre who trained before work-hour limitations (before Libby Zion) and their younger counterparts who are now entering practice and never worked 30 hours at a stretch on a ward. The former roll their eyes quietly when a trainee leaves rounds at the end of his "shift" and, when talking privately, bemoan the end of the "days of the giants." Giants didn't do *shifts*. Younger doctors, on the other hand, hear "giant" and think "giant dinosaur."

To this day, the exact cause of Libby Zion's death remains unclear. She was undoubtedly sicker than the doctors who cared for her appreciated. Legitimate questions have been raised about why she wasn't visited by a doctor as she became more and more agitated during the wee hours of that fateful Monday morning. She should not have been given a drug that was, in the medical vernacular, "contraindicated" because of its potential for interaction with the antidepressant she had taken. But Libby's symptoms of fever and agitation were present before she got the contraindicated dose of Demerol. Luise Weinstein shouldn't have prescribed the drug; but, she actually had gone to the trouble of reading through an encyclopedia of drugs and checking for interactions before she wrote the order. She just missed this *one* item in reading the small type. Today's computerized systems would have warned her of the drug-to-drug interaction and might have prevented the error.

As the details of Zion's death became public, largely through the efforts of Sydney Zion, those of us who were still in medical training at the time spent a lot amount of time thinking and talking about the case. The general consensus was: "There, but for the grace of God, go I." We all knew what it was like to be up admitting a patient at three in the morning. It wasn't easy, but you actually don't feel tired then; the mind-numbing fatigue sets in much later.

The fact that Weinstein had missed a drug interaction described in the *Physicians' Desk Reference* wasn't surprising to any of us. That's like missing a "begat" in the Bible: both books weigh about the same, have about the same number of words and typically share the same diminutive type size. In fact, as we followed the Libby Zion story, most of us gave the intern extra credit for even checking for drug interactions in the first place.

The 1980s-era medical community concluded that there was nothing particularly egregious about the care Libby Zion received that night and that the whole issue of work hours, as depicted in the press at the time, had become a scapegoat. The term *scapegoat* actually derives from the book of Leviticus in the Bible, in which a goat is driven into the wilderness, metaphorically carrying off the sins of the people. Scapegoat has latterly come to refer to something or someone that is innocent and yet blamed, and punished, for the sins of others, typically acting as a distraction from the real cause.

If a medical error had indeed been responsible for Libby's fever and subsequent cardiac arrest, we knew it wasn't fundamentally a house-staff sleep problem, and we knew our residencies were being blamed and punished as a result of some displaced or misplaced anger on the part of Sydney Zion. Of course, that was the view from the inside out. In a sense, we residents of the 1980s were all suffering from a variant of the Stockholm syndrome, the term deriving from a 1973 hostage incident in Sweden in which the hostages came to identify with their captors after several days of captivity and eventually actually resisted rescue attempts.

Through Sydney Zion's efforts, the outside world got a peek at the real working conditions of a modern medical resident, and it was appalled. To the viewers, once the gritty details were revealed, it was as if someone had suddenly told them that their running shoes were being put together by enslaved children in Southeast Asia. The sneakers were fine as long as one didn't know about the sweathouses in which they were assembled—just as patients were fine with medical care being provided by tired house officers in the idealized Kildare and Casey mold, but not so fine with it when they saw the conditions in which Luise Weinstein and Gregg Stone worked at a flagship academic medical center. And they were most definitely *not* fine when someone suggested that a tired doctor might screw up their care or kill them. With that observation, change essentially became inevitable.

It took a very short period of time after work hours rules went into effect before residents' expectations of their life during residency changed. Residency programs developed coverage grids showing exactly when residents were expected to be at the hospital and when they were expected to leave. Hospitals hired nurse practitioners and physician assistants to fill in any gaps in the work day. Call schedules went from one in three nights "in house" to one in four. Residents suddenly had predictable days off, and they could say with assurance to spouses or potential spouses, partners, dentists or hairdressers, that they would be free at a given date and time. They knew that there were mechanisms in place to hand off patient care regardless of what was going on at the time. If a complication developed in the midst of an operation, it was now understood that the resident might still need to leave at some designated witching hour. The operation, of course, would go on.

In short, residents' lives went from being largely uncontrollable to pretty predictable, more or less overnight. They "got a life." The culture of training hospitals changed quickly. As the duration of stretches in the hospital became better defined, with predetermined start- and end-points, residencies began to move away from the relatively formless apprenticeship model to something structured more like professional school with prescribed periods of shift work.

This new model was no longer years of training in which work alternated with periods of sleep; it became one in which there were predictable intervals of work, sleep and *discretionary time*. In fact, the discretionary time became so predictable that residents no longer saw any reason to put their "real" lives on hold during their training. Once unheard of, it became routine for female residents to take pregnancy leave. And, as we saw in the email that I cited at the beginning of the chapter, an occasional resident even saw fit to integrate a time-critical procedure such as in vitro fertilization into a mission-critical rotation in the intensive care unit.

This move to a more-balanced lifestyle for medical trainees was long overdue. The slavish conditions revealed by the Bell commission were not designed to be so; medicine had just become increasingly complex and all-consuming during the course of the twentieth century, and medical trainees got sucked along in the slipstream. The model had to change at some point, and the Libby Zion incident served as a convincing punctuation point. The days of the giants were indeed over. But with the passage of the giants, something else changed—something largely unspoken, but something traditionalists believe will change the nature of the doctor-patient relationship forever.

The culture of medicine in the era of the giants was one in which doctors put the lives of their patients before their own. Physicians would miss the birth of their children because they were "tied up in the operating room." They weren't home when the kids were sick. They missed grade-school graduations and birthday parties. They got up in the middle of the night to deliver babies. They went to work sick. Certain residency programs were described as being so tough that "no resident's marriage survived the internship year." Self-sacrifice and spousal sacrifice were the norm, in part because young physicians were steeped in that environment from the first days of their training. Today's young physicians train in what most of us would consider to be a much saner world, but it is a world in which their own lives are given equal priority to that of their patients. For better or worse, it is, as we'll see, no longer a world in which the physician will drop whatever he or she is doing to rush to the side of his or her patient.

PART III

NEW METHODS OF CARE

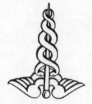

As medicine's pace becomes faster and faster and we gather more information about diseases and their victims, we're outstripping the abilities of our providers to keep up. And one clear lesson is that data begets data. We're about to enter an era in which we'll all have a copy of our own personal owner's manual—our genome—that will open a Pandora's box of new information. The digitization of information and the automation of decision making will become inevitable; no human can keep up any longer.

In the third section of the book, we'll look over the shoulder of my father as he scrawls out notes about his patients in a distinctive yet indecipherable scrawl. And we'll compare his notes to those in an emerging generation of electronic medical records. We'll see how computers have begun to automate certain types of medical care and analysis, freeing up their warm-blooded owners to do the things that humans do best. We'll watch how medical care will take flight through the airwaves, allowing doctors to reach out across great distances. And we'll meet computers and robots that can analyze their environment and make certain kinds of medical decisions based on what they see and know.

CHAPTER 10

BINOCULAR VISION

I grew up in a household where the word "dictation" had special resonance. Although my father wasn't a dictator, he *was* a slave to dictation—not my mother's—because he had to dictate to communicate medical information. Dad was a general practitioner with really bad handwriting, so bad in fact that the letters I got from him—back before email, texting and social media—were very nearly unintelligible. They were always signed "Love, Dad," which was what really mattered, but I could only make out occasional frustrating glimpses of his chatty stories and questions.

On a first encounter with a new patient, my father would focus mainly on his impressions and what he heard from the patient. He'd sit in the exam room, occasionally scribbling on a large index card a word, a quote or a thought, like: "67 yo," "tachypneic" (short of breath), "cough," "can only walk up a few steps," "only at night!" and "jugular venous distension." Based on these short notes, he might later construct a case for early heart failure. He used a variety of elegant gold or black fountain pens, and each had some mechanism, like a bulb or piston, with which one could suck ink into its internal reservoir. He preferred inks like Parker's Black Quink brand or Sheaffer's Blue-Black Skrip. The ink was messy and "permanent"; although I loved to help with pen filling, I invariably ended up with blue or black stains on my fingers that took a few days to wear off.

I came across a box of his old medical records several years after his death and in it found reams of paper with spidery writing walking across the card at odd angles, sometimes even up and down the margins. He was left-handed, and unlike some of his contemporaries, was never forced to convert to right-handed penmanship. Lefties are at a significant handicap when writing English—as opposed to writing Chinese, for example, which runs from top to bottom—because they are constantly covering up what they've just written as the left hand moves from left to right across the page. Their difficulties are exacerbated when the writer uses a fountain pen, because fountain ink doesn't dry as quickly or spread as evenly as inks from modern pens. The left-handed fountain-pen writer has to find some way to write around his writing, lest he smear it; and many fountain pen nibs are designed to be used by righties.

In fact the whole "problem" of *sinistrality*, or left-handedness, and penmanship was the subject of a 1939 publication entitled "Instruction in Penmanship for the Left-Handed Child," written by a Luella Cole for the *Elementary School Journal* in 1939.[1] Ms. Cole's motivation is clearly benevolent. As she puts it,

> The first and most obvious source of difficulty has nothing to do with the actual technique of writing. It is purely emotional. From his first day in school a left-handed child is subject to pressure. Both parents and teachers bewail his condition. They may encourage him to use his right hand. Even though nothing is said to him on this point, he may insist on trying to be right-handed....If he succeeds in his attempt, he escapes from the nagging criticism—overt or implied—that is the normal lot of the sinistral, but he subjects himself to intense and continued nervous strain. Let any right-handed person who doubts the existence of this strain resolutely write with his left hand for a month; he will gain some insight into the chronic nervous exhaustion that accompanies any effort to alter inborn eye-hand co-ordinations.

In her tract, Ms. Cole says of the sinistrals: "Six years from now most of them will emerge from elementary school using handwriting which is barely legible and which is produced awkwardly and at the cost of unreasonable effort." She suggests that the teacher "must begin by altering her own feeling that a left-handed pupil is a nuisance," and that the student will consequently no longer be "uncomfortable under the emotional pressure of being considered queer."

Aside from the issue that I pointed out about smeared ink, Cole notes the tendency for paper to "walk from under the hand" of the sinistral as he writes, because he's not as able to pin down the paper with his forearm as a righty is; she also refers to the southpaw's need to push rather than pull the tip of the implement, be it pencil or pen, the consequent perforations of the paper, and ink blobs, and so on.

My father's scrawls would scream "lefty" to a handwriting analyst at a single glance. While writing, he adopted a characteristic wrap-around technique, one of several potential compensations for sinistrality noted by Ms. Cole. His left hand and arm would curl around the paper from above so that he was, in effect, writing upside down, at least from his hand's perspective. And as he wrapped, his arm was consequently foreshortened, which pulled his head closer to the page. In order to read the slanted script from this near-sighted position, he had to tilt his head at an odd angle. To me, a righty, the whole thing all looked pretty physically uncomfortable. We never did get around to talking about whether or not it was emotionally distressing, as Ms. Cole suggests, because there were lots of other issues to cover when we had face time. As I think about this today, I guess Ms. Cole's nice suggestions in her *Elementary School Journal* piece are the 1930s equivalent of our own modern ruminations about the emotional consequences of sexting and cyber-bullying.

"Instruction in Penmanship for the Left-Handed Child" includes suggestions for positioning the paper, gripping the pen, positioning the hand relative to the baseline, slanting the script and selecting the correct writing implement. The last sentence of her thesis reads: "Let every teacher realize that *any* legible writing which is produced without strain is good writing." Cole's fundamental message is that good penmanship results in effective and efficient communication, a standard my father's medical records completely failed to meet. He was, however, writing primarily for himself. He would scribble his notes while the patient was in the room or just after she'd left, and only much later, being a world-class procrastinator, use them to dictate the information into some more generally accessible format for communication to others.

Growing up, I sensed that dictation was like penance for him, and that the word had the same guilt-ridden, shameful feelings we've all had about whatever it is we wish we could manage better—be it paying bills, doing laundry, staying healthy or staying in touch. That observation probably played a significant role in steering me toward a specialty in medicine in which I never, ever have to dictate—anesthesiologists record their encounters while they're caring for their patients.

There *were* good aspects to Dad's dictation, however, because he'd usually take one or more of us kids along to the hospital on a weekend morning while he droned out a bunch of letters into the Dictaphone. We'd play with his fluoroscope (an office-based x-ray machine), otoscope (the ear examination tool), blood pressure cuff or ophthalmoscope and careen around the office having wheelchair jousts. I learned how to use these instruments at the same age that ranch-raised kids learn how to ride a horse or throw a lariat.

My father was in a group practice that operated on a fee-for-service basis, and he employed a small staff that handled billing, scheduling, phone calls and his endless dictation. They'd take tapes that he had dictated using his portable or desktop recorder and feed them into a transcription machine equipped with a headset and a pedal control that allowed them to use foot movements to navigate back and forth through the material while they typed. Then they transcribed his oral notes, typing them onto what was called onionskin paper that would replace his handwritten notes in the medical record. Office practices no longer use employed transcriptionists today; the transcription function is handled by speech-recognition software or outsourced to large, often international companies.

Dad's transcribed records were his personal medical chart. The aggregate transcription, correspondence and lab results were stored in folders in file cabinets scattered about the offices used by the three doctors in his practice. At some later point, the hanging folders with the patient names typed on tabs were replaced by folders with a color-coded sequence of tape on one end that allowed a secretary to quickly scan a cabinet full of records for the right patient. These manila folders were like party dresses: they were colorful and held lots of secrets but spent most of their time hanging in the closet. Of course, as with party dresses, some people's folders saw a lot more action than others.

A doctor's private medical records didn't travel back then. In a very real sense, medical records represented the "intellectual property" of a typical general practitioner. In fact, these records were a major component of the thing one physician historically transferred to another when she sold her practice. As an indication of how precious this information can be, I know of one situation in which an alert physician raided the patient files of another within hours of the latter's sudden death. The raider culled his dead colleague's medical records of choice patients, contacted them and let them know of his interest in assuming their care.

There's a word used in medicine to describe flat, immobile tumors, like warts. The same word, *sessile,* is also used in biology to describe plants or animals that are permanently attached to some feature in the landscape, as barnacles are to a piling. Like many English words, the word sessile has ancient roots: it actually comes from the Latin root word meaning "stunted," which is a pretty good way of describing medical information that is permanently attached to a file cabinet in some doctor's private office. Paper records like my father's were sessile, with stunted possibilities. And the vast majority of medical records in most doctors' offices in most countries in the world are still paper. As a result, most medical care is predicated on the limitations inherent in various forms of sessile medical information like office charts, hospital charts and correspondence. These are all one-off copies of critical information, typically unavailable when needed for the patient who arrives in the emergency room with an acute medical problem.

There are some definite benefits to paper records. Their relative immobility makes it less likely that they will be viewed by the wrong eyes, so they are arguably more secure. Paper records also give the recorder—the nurse or physician—more latitude in characterizing patient encounters. However unscientific, a note saying "She looks SMASHING today!" scrawled in a big, black-inked hand, has a certain charm and conveys information a computer record could never duplicate. So does an entry to the effect that "Mrs. Smith seems a bit more lethargic today," like one fabled handwritten note that was said to have immediately followed another indicating that Mrs. Smith had been pronounced dead 20 minutes earlier. But the charms of paper records don't even begin to counterbalance downsides relating to their perishability, illegibility and inaccessibility, and the inconsistency of the paper itself, when compared to their computerized equivalent—which is why the United States government put $20 billion on the table to enhance adoption of electronic health records in the 2009 Health Information Technology for Economic and Clinical Health Act.

The biggest, and an often unnoted, drawback to paper records is that they promote the practice of provincial medicine. A physician like my father, who recorded his interactions with patients on paper charts and kept them in his own filing cabinets, could very well have begun his career using practices that remained unaltered and uninformed by advances in medicine for the rest of his 40-odd-year career. It was almost impossible for him to compare his management of common diseases like hypertension or diabetes to that of colleagues in the next hallway, much less across the country or world. To be sure, there were published studies of specific practices and drugs, but studies of a drug, disease or technique are not always directly relevant to the day-to-day management of a patient.

In fact, today's doctors often have very different ways of managing exactly the same problem. And if we were to take a giant slice through your average medical arts building full of general practitioners, each with their set of medical records in sequestered file cabinets, we'd uncover something very like a hill full of moles. Adjacent doctors would certainly be aware of their neighbors through encounters in corridors and by the occasional muffled exclamation from the next suite, but they'd be as blind to each other's interactions with patients as if they all lived underground.

For some, this represents a blessing because there's nothing beautiful about the way they practice. Others, however, practice elegantly, effectively and efficiently but never get a chance to shine. Someday soon, the era of paper records will be regarded as an era of subterranean medicine, and the coming era of the electronic health record will be one in which, for better and for worse, medical practices come stumbling into the light.

The evolutionary origins of vision have been traced back to a primitive organism related to jellyfish, coral and sea anemones. The hydra is actually a small, predatory freshwater animal, only a few millimeters long. It has concentrations of light-sensitive proteins called *opsins* around its mouth and was the earliest animal to show signs of sight 600 million years ago. The modern hydra has up to 12 tentacles that sweep food toward the mouth, and the tentacles are equipped with stinging cells that fire neurotoxin-containing-darts into prey.

Flatworms came along later and developed simple eyespots. In subsequent evolutionary steps, the eyespot recessed into a cup for protection, and the cup has the added benefit of allowing the localization of a light source. With time, the eyespot retracted further into the cup and developed a transparent cover to shield the light-sensitive layer, which eventually evolved into a lens. Along the way, new or nearby muscles serving other purposes were brought to bear to steer the eye and change the relationship between the lens and the retina and change the eye's focal length.

During the course of this remarkable evolution, the eye became attached to the evolving brain via the optic nerve. This sequence of steps describes the evolution of the "camera eye" of the mammal and squid; alternate visual mechanisms have emerged in insects like the fly, which has a spherical compound eye.

Vision conveys special advantages to the sighted, such as an enhanced ability to find food or mates, to avoid predators and to explore the environment. The evolutionary advantages of vision are so compelling that eyes have evolved independently in at least 40 different groups of animals.

The eye ultimately serves as an extremely efficient mechanism to bring information from a distance to the attention of an animal. Consider the eyesight of the owl, a sometimes nocturnal hunter that can see an object that's half a mile away and lit merely by a candle. The internet, too, has given us the ability to see information from afar, and the electronic health record will act like an eye in the medical care of the future, gathering and focusing data so that the right information is available to the right stakeholder—be it provider or patient—in the right format, through the right electronic vehicle, at the right time.

When my father interacted with his medical records, his field of view was confined to the exam room. He was able to see what he had written previously and any labs that had come in since the last visit, assuming his secretarial staff had filed them in the chart. He might have letters from referring or corresponding physicians. The patient would offer whatever information she could, in the form of her complaints and physical examination. But that was it. Dad's senses were pretty much confined to that room, as if he were underground like a mole. Some doctors today, and all doctors tomorrow, will be able to see through the eyes of the electronic health record, which shouldn't be thought of as merely a computerized version of the old paper chart but as something that will serve as a real-time, two-way portal to the much larger medical world.

Using some of today's, already soon-to-be-antiquated, electronic health records, a doctor or nurse working in, for example, a medical arts building or a hospital can access any patient's record from any terminal at any time, assuming they have access rights. In fact, multiple people can access the same chart simultaneously—an impossibility with a paper record—allowing the doctor to review a chart before seeing a patient that the nurse is prepping in another room. Information from a patient's visits to other physicians can be available. Lab tests and x-rays may be integrated into the record. Abnormal results may be automatically highlighted. And some of these systems allow the doctor to access up-to-the-minute information about a test, a medication or the best-practice management of a disease like diabetes or hypertension.

These capabilities represent dramatic advances over the way my father practiced and allow the practitioner to begin to "see" information from the world outside of his examination room, in real-time. But these first-generation electronic medical records should also be thought of as analogous to those very primitive first-generation eyespots on a flatworm—essentially as precursor eyes for the medical profession.

I work in what's considered to be a well-wired health system; we are advanced users of information technology. We use electronic health records in our outpatient clinics, in our emergency ward, on hospital floors and in the intensive care units. I use these tools regularly, and they are an infinite improvement over the old paper record for a whole host of reasons.

First, I can always find the record when I need to, merely by logging in to the nearest computer. Not *all* of our floors are computerized, and when I'm on an *un*wired floor, it may take me several minutes to find a patient's paper chart. When I do, it may be in the hands of some other doctor who is off in an alcove reading it while munching her lunch. When I do finally get the paper record, the entries may be as illegible as my father's were; whereas his records were mainly for his own consumption, the hospital charts are meant to be information vehicles for all providers.

Our electronic records, on the other hand, are always legible. Most of the electronic charts that I use automatically provide up-to-the minute information about laboratory studies that I can reference while I am reviewing the record. But, for all of our advances, we use different brands of electronic records in each location, and they don't all talk to one another very well. The emergency room system, for example, doesn't at all communicate well with the outpatient electronic record, except in what amounts to "pidgin" computer. As a result, the clinician who tries to piece together an image of the whole patient, even using relatively advanced systems like ours, has to work with a group of picture fragments from each of the location-specific electronic systems augmented in some cases by paper records. As with flatworms' eyes, today's records give some vision, but don't really let the doctor see a coherent picture.

Interestingly, some of today's more advanced electronic record systems do allow us to see an actual, live picture of the patient. For example, when I work with our electronic intensive care system, I can click an icon and access a kind of a webcam that allows me to see the patient and zoom in on her, her data monitors and other equipment in her room to see what's going on. The same electronic system also allows me to write an electronic note about what I see and think. I can see the results of laboratory studies as they are completed. The system alerts me about abnormal laboratory values or vital signs. And I can electronically flip through notes from the other doctors and nurses caring for that patient. I can even look up the state-of-the-art approach to the management of a rare medical condition that I might otherwise have to review in a book.

This same audiovisual capability is beginning to be deployed in home-care systems for elderly or chronically ill patients. These home-based systems can measure patients' blood pressure, record their weight and laboratory studies—like home glucose tests for diabetics. Smart software embedded in the equipment in the home can analyze this data and look for troublesome results or trends, and, if necessary, alert both the patient and a provider. If appropriate, a two-way audiovisual link can be established to permit a direct conversation between the two: "Mrs. Jones, your blood pressure appears to be elevated, are you taking your blood pressure medication regularly?"

Medical knowledge has grown so quickly and changes so rapidly that it is no longer realistic to commit every disease, drug and practice to memory, so online access to best-practice management is tremendously helpful. All of these capabilities can be thought of as developmental steps in medicine's evolution of vision. And each incremental step provides a fitness advantage to the "partially sighted"—early technology adopter—doctor over his blind colleague.

The intern of yore had to call the laboratory, go find x-rays, transcribe medical information from one chart to another, and onto index cards, and so on. She was constantly on the move just as Luise Weinstein had been the night she was trying to look after Libby Zion and a host of other patients. Her contemporary counterpart can manage all of this much more efficiently without leaving her assigned floor, by using electronic records.

But our medical "vision" is still extremely primitive. Most American doctors don't have access to any electronic health record. A study published in the *New England Journal* in 2009 found that only 1.5 percent of U.S. hospitals had a comprehensive records system present in all units, and 7.5 percent had a basic system that was operative in at least one clinical unit. The adoption of electronic records in doctor's offices that are not based in a hospital is similarly low. By contrast, nearly all hospitals in the Netherlands have a comprehensive system. Even if a physician in the United States does use some form of electronic record, his vision is very near-sighted, because current computerized records only provide a fragmentary picture of a patient's total lifelong medical experience.

Gennifer Florez has been followed for years in one of our outpatient practices for diabetes and high blood pressure. She's an overweight, 45-year-old mother of teenagers, and she spends a lot of time running around getting the kids from one place to another or doing what we euphemistically describe as "the activities of daily living." Her finances have been tight recently because her husband lost his job as a cable company repairman. The family's health care is covered by Medicaid, but she admits she doesn't take good care of herself: "I don't have the time."

Gennifer has been seen intermittently at her doctor's office, one of the few with its own electronic records. Her visits there are maintained in a system that's customized for outpatient encounters, allowing her doctor to see labs, send secure messages to colleagues, write prescriptions and keep running notes from each visit. This system is great for continuity between visits, but a problem came up on the day when she had her heart problem.

Gennifer was late and stuck in traffic while trying to pick her daughter up from the high school after a social event. She knew that Tina didn't have her cell phone with her because when she'd tried calling her earlier, the phone rang in the girl's bedroom. This was an unprecedented lapse, both because she'd insisted Tina be available by cell whenever she was out and also because the girl seemed to live on Facebook—using the phone as a communication link to the social media site. She also knew her daughter would be standing outside the school in a bad neighborhood waiting for her in the dark.

Traffic wasn't moving. She had no way to get in touch with her daughter. Her anxiety kept mounting. As she told us later, the last thing she felt before passing out was a "clutching sensation" in her throat. When her car stopped traffic, an angry, then anxious, driver found her slumped over the wheel and quickly called 9-1-1. With the help of other drivers, one of whom had been trained in Advanced Cardiac Life Support, she was pulled from the car, laid on the ground and cardiopulmonary resuscitation was started almost immediately.

Gennifer was taken to our emergency department where we have our own, very sophisticated, homegrown electronic medical records, specially designed for emergency encounters. Unfortunately, these records don't yet communicate with the outpatient records in which information from Gennifer's previous encounters were stored. So the ER doctors had to work more or less from scratch to gather her medical information, including the many risk factors she had for what turned out to be a "silent heart attack," something that sometimes happens in younger women with diabetes. The emergency doctors dutifully entered all of Gennifer's information into her ER record that everyone in the ER would use to collaboratively enter and view data during her stay—which was brief because she was whisked up to the cardiac catheterization suite where they discovered the blockages in her coronary arteries.

Our cardiology catheterization systems have their own specialty electronic records customized for the kind of information that's very specific to patients with heart disease. These systems, created by companies specializing in cardiology software, were designed for patients with cardiac problems. Gennifer's coronary artery blockages were diagnosed and treated immediately. The blocked sections were dilated using a technique known as *balloon angioplasty,* in which a balloon is expanded at the site of a narrowing in a blood vessel, thereby expanding it to its normal, pre-disease caliber. Special metal stents, which slowly release immunosuppressant drugs to prevent the cell growth that causes coronary plaques, were then positioned across the diseased area, acting both structurally and chemically to prevent re-blockage.

Eventually the cardiology folks decided that Gennifer needed to be admitted to our intensive care unit, which has its own specially designed electronic record. As you might have guessed, it doesn't talk to her outpatient electronic record or the emergency department record or the cardiology record. So the intensive care doctors had to start over and reenter, yet again, all of her history and related information. After a while, Gennifer got better and was discharged to the floor, which has *its* own computerized record.

The bottom line is that we have a lot of computerized records in our hospital, which puts us way ahead of a lot of other institutions, but these component "eyes" only give us a limited picture of our patients, very much like the one you might have of yourself if you looked into a frame full of mirror fragments.

Our computer records aren't well integrated today. Primitive eyes weren't either. But eventually the eyes became more sophisticated, synchronized, steerable and focusable. Some eyes, like those of the eagle, conferred their owner with the ability to see great distances. The electronic health record will eventually mature into an instrument with all the capabilities of an advanced eye, permitting a general practitioner to efficiently scan a large amount of data on a single patient, looking through a lifetime's worth of medical information much like an owl scans for food from the sky. An epidemiologist might scan data from a large population of patients, looking for individuals with certain characteristics, like the lioness who scans a herd of gazelles, looking for the weak ones.

This same electronic eye will be capable of closely focusing in on an important minutia, like the heart rate for a specific hour of a hospitalization; or of zooming out to see the blood pressure trend over a year. As the electronic record becomes ubiquitous, it won't matter that a patient was seen at another hospital or doctor's office, perhaps across the world, because all records will have become integrated and we'll be able to see all of them from far off. This same integrative process occurred in the banking industry over two decades ago.

I distinctly remember standing outside a bank somewhere in the wine country north of San Francisco one day shortly after I had moved from Pennsylvania to Palo Alto's Stanford University Medical Center to begin a residency. I still maintained a bank account on the East Coast at that time and had forgotten to bring cash with me on this day trip. Automated teller machines were slowly becoming prevalent at that point, but most of the ATMs were only connected to a few localized "interbank networks."

I had this eureka moment when I walked up to a machine and saw that it was connected across country to the same network as my eastern bank. The memory of the crisp new twenties rolling out of that machine's dispenser has stuck with me ever since, as a tectonic shift in my personal banking life. That same ATM let me see how much money I had on deposit in a bank thousands of miles away. Today, of course, I can get on a plane to Istanbul with a pocket full of change, fully confident that I can get a fistful of Turkish lira drawn from my bank account and dispensed by a teller machine in the city's 550-year-old Grand Bazaar—to buy a Persian rug perhaps. In the not-too-distant future, a doctor on one side of the world will be able to see the medical information of a tourist from the other side of the world, with the same degree of transparency and security.

Our paired, binocular eyes permit depth perception, and medical devices will soon give us a three-, or four-, and even many-dimensional view of our health, channeling multiple streams of interrelated data essential to medical diagnosis, treatment and health maintenance. Like the always-open eyes of the housefly, the electronic medical record and linked medical devices, like one's cell phone, will eventually become perpetually vigilant and warn the doctor, or a proxy, whenever trouble is brewing. Eventually, critical information will be accessible on your primary doctor's smartphone or desktop that may have originated from your smartphone or from your home health system or from a consultant, a laboratory or a radiology system that knows something important about you. Medical information will be connected electronically from one end to the other, like so many of today's information infrastructures in other industries.

There will be a comprehensive conduit of medical information not dissimilar to today's social media networks: constantly updated and ubiquitous. As with social media, medical networks will eventually evolve to permit continuous bi-directional communication. In fact, it's possible that the medical record of the future will ultimately come to look like a Facebook page, controlled by the patient but with permissions granted to doctors and hospitals to post information.

This would be a radical departure from the paradigm of the past in which doctors, like my father, and hospitals controlled the medical records of their patients. Whatever form the computerized records of the future take, there will inevitably be a greater degree of two-way exchange and transparency between the doctor and the patient, with the electronic health record as the conduit.

The doctor of the future will use the electronic record as his eyes. These eyes will provide him with the ability to see his patient's data, to access information essential to his practice—perhaps even to see his patient directly. Certain doctors have already specialized and evolved to fill the new ecological niches created by the development, care and maintenance of electronic charts. These medical informaticians are physicians or nurses who design tools specifically to enhance the workflow of clinicians or to format data in a way that enhances the ability of a provider to recognize problems. And informaticians design computerized decision-support tools, about which we'll talk more in the next chapter. Computerized decision support tools are intended to provide doctors with exactly the right information at the right time to improve patient care. Just as the development of sight provided species with such an evolutionary advantage that it has evolved over and over again in different species, the development of electronic records will result in medical evolutionary advances we can't yet imagine.

Gennifer Florez eventually left the hospital after her heart attack. Her coronary arteries had been replumbed, and her daughter Tina pushed her wheelchair from the hospital floor all the way to her husband's car where he idled in the hospital's carport. (Tina had waited outside her school on that fateful night for about half an hour before finally, and safely, catching a ride home with a friend. It was only on her arrival there that she found out what had happened to her mother.)

There's nothing to suggest that Gennifer's heart attack would have been treated any differently if there had been interconnected electronic records. Nonetheless, the significant inefficiencies in her care did have ramifications. The same medical information was reentered repeatedly into different systems by different providers, which wastes the time of busy doctors and nurses. Inefficiency is a common complaint from patients, too. They are forced to repeat the same history over and over during the course of a hospitalization, which is increasingly irksome in world where Google and Amazon seem to already know everything about us, without a single interview, and can present individually tailored advertisements or shopping suggestions regardless of where or how one logs in.

CHAPTER 11

KNEE JERK

While the Gross Anatomy rotation is perhaps the most well-known initiation rite into the mysteries of medicine for the acolyte, there is another class to which medical students look forward with perhaps even a greater degree of fear and trepidation. Physical Diagnosis was the class in which I first learned to violate another individual's intimate space—to move in close enough to smell her breath and the sweat on her body, and for her to smell mine.

A skilled physician's examination actually starts the moment she encounters a new patient, whether he be sitting in a chair, lying on a bed or walking down a hallway—and well before she ever lays on a hand. Does the patient look older or younger than he claims? What is the texture of his face, hair and skin? What does his body language say? Does he make eye contact? How much does he weigh?

All of this information flows into the doctor's brain, where it is processed against an accumulated database of past encounters—essentially without any conscious thought. Watch a doctor the next time he watches you. This first impression is his Gestalt—a body of information so unified and coherent that it exceeds the sum of its separate elements. With this background, and informed by a store of experience, the diagnostician then sets about a systematic verbal and physical examination designed to screen for problems or diseases.

The physical exam typically starts with the patient's head, ears, eyes, nose and throat. The hearing can be tested with tuning forks at low and high frequencies. The movements of the eyes and the pupil's reactions to light can be tested without special equipment; examination of the retina requires facility with the portable ophthalmoscope.

The whites of the eyes, the lips, the tongue and the nail beds all act like semi-opaque windows on the inner workings of the body. A skilled medical eye can distinguish the quick from the soon-to-be dead with a mere glance at these membranes. The throat contains the thyroid gland, important lymph nodes and the brain's big source vessels, the carotids. The head's posture speaks volumes about a patient's personality; there's world of different between the aggressive forward thrust of the Type A, heart-attack-waiting-to-happen, and the slumped head and rolled shoulders of the perpetually submissive.

The emphysematous smoker has a barrel chest that resonates like a kettle drum when it's struck with a stiffened, percussing finger, and the nuances of the cardiac examination are the subjects of full textbooks. There's the normal *lub-dub* we're all familiar with, as well as a whole variety of whooshes, squeaks, and rubbing and burring sounds indicating problems of one sort or another. The belly contains big important items like the liver, kidney, spleen and the bowels, and the deft examiner can identify many big problems by the look, sound and feel of these organs.

While necessary, the genital and rectal exams are the most invasive part of a comprehensive evaluation. They provide the examiner with an admittedly uncomfortable way to feel deeply seated organs like the man's prostate or the woman's cervix and uterus. Prior to the development of sophisticated dummies, medical students learned how to do pelvic and rectal examinations on volunteer model patients. I remember the awkwardness of performing a pelvic exam on a live "model" who told me that I wasn't really feeling her ovary *there*, and that I actually needed to move my hand *here*.

But the brain and nervous system are what animate the patient—putting the sparkle in the eye, the spring in the step and the words in the mouth—absent which a human being is a slack-limbed, empty jumble of meat and bones. Reflexes are tested as part of the neurological survey during the physical exam.

The reflex hammer comes in many shapes. The one I carried in residency had a triangular, red rubber hammer at one end, and at the other a sharp metal tip with which we test a comatose patient's reflexive response to pain by stroking the point up the sole of the foot. Even a severely brain-damaged patient will pull a limb reflexively away from a painful stimulus like this. Reflexes are a primitive but almost universal adaptation found throughout the animal kingdom, and they allow an organism to maintain its equilibrium and defend itself. As we'll see, the same streamlined components that nature uses in designing reflexes will soon be used to enhance the safety and efficiency of patient care.

The knee-jerk reflex is one of the signature elements of the physical exam. To perform this test, we were taught to have the patient (and in our class this was one of our fellow students) sit on the side of a table with his knees dangling freely over the side. The legs had to be relaxed for the test to work, and the examiner has to strike the patellar tendon, which attaches the kneecap to the shinbone, very precisely; the reflex doesn't work as well when you hit the kneecap or the shin, and it only annoys the patient.

The knee-jerk reflex, and any other reflex for that matter, demonstrate the body's way of responding very rapidly to potentially dangerous situations. For example, we pull our finger reflexively away from a hot surface even before the sensation of "hot" ever reaches the brain. This reflex response takes much less time than it would to form the following thought process: "Oops. I have just touched something really hot that will hurt my skin. I need to contract my biceps muscle and get my finger as far away as possible from that hot thing as quickly as I can." The human body is actually wired for thousands of protective or bodily maintenance reflexes, ranging from the very simple knee-jerk circuit to much more sophisticated reflexes involving many parts of the nervous system as well as the organs and muscles it controls. While it looks impressive, the knee-jerk reflex really only consists of four elements.

When the patellar tendon is struck, a specialized structure called a *muscle spindle*, which is embedded in the quadriceps muscle of the thigh, detects the stretching force as the patella is pulled downward by the hammer blow. Muscle spindles, which are also called *stretch receptors*, consist of specialized muscle cells embedded throughout all skeletal muscle. The spindle's job is to keep the brain informed about the position of a muscle. These specialized sensors are designed to help maintain posture as well as to prevent muscles from becoming overstretched and torn apart.

One of the reasons a now-discredited method of gym class stretching—the one where you bend over and bounce your fingers toward your toes—never works is that with every bounce the muscle spindles activate and "fire," which actually causes the hamstring to contract rather than to lengthen, which is obviously counterproductive. Similarly, the knee-jerk reflex works as follows. When the patellar tendon is struck by the hammer, the quadriceps muscle is stretched sharply, and, in response, its spindles "fire" a signal to the spinal cord, a foot or two away, via a *sensory* nerve. A signaling chemical called *glutamate* is released within the spinal cord, causing a linked *motor* nerve to send a message immediately back down to the muscle—without checking in with the brain—telling it to contract "reflexively." The knee jerks in response. This automatic reflex is hard-wired and essentially impossible to override. And while this knee-jerk reflex may sound complicated, it is actually controlled by a very simple nerve circuit consisting of a *sensor* muscle spindle, two nerves and an *effector*, which is, in this case, the quadriceps muscle. We will soon use these same design elements to improve medical care using electronic logic.

I meet with many of my patients before their heart surgery, and one of the most common questions I get is: "Will I be awake on the respirator after the operation?" This may be accompanied by some variant of: "My cousin Vinnie was and he gagged for hours." Patients know about this unpleasantness and don't want to be on "the machine" any longer than necessary. We used to give heart surgery patients very high doses of anesthesia that kept them asleep overnight, and everyone got taken off the respirator first thing the next morning. Recent research, however, has shown that there are lots of good reasons to shorten the time on the machine as much as possible. In fact, most good ICUs have protocols that accelerate what we call *ventilator weaning*, the process by which we slowly lessen machine support while allowing the patient to take over. These protocols have helped to reduce this period to a matter of a few hours, but the humans often slow down the process.

David McCaslin had an abnormal aortic heart valve. A cross-section of that valve is normally shaped like the Mercedes-Benz logo. It has three leaflets that open with each beat of the heart, allowing blood to flow out, and then they flap back into position to prevent reflow. McCaslin's valve, however, had only two leaflets, and its cross-section looked more like a Cheshire smile. The problem with having this kind of abnormal "bicuspid," or two-leafed, valve is that its leaflets often stiffen over time, forcing the heart to work harder to get blood into circulation. The three-leaflet valve is the one nature prefers. As is often the case with bi-leaflet valves, McCaslin had developed heart failure and required an artificial replacement heart valve.

When I talked to him before the operation, David looked up at me from his recumbent position on the operating room table and asked me how long it would be until he was awake and could talk to his family once the surgery was through. Patients are in a pretty vulnerable position on a narrow OR bed, and we'd just read him the long lists of risks associated with the operation, including stroke and death. I knew he was asking more than just: "What time will I wake up?" He really wanted the answer that he *would* wake up, with no hint of *if*.

This was at 7 o'clock in the morning, just before I put him to sleep for the operation using a combination of anesthetics. I told him I anticipated he'd start coming out of the anesthesia early in the afternoon, assuming the operation went smoothly, and that the breathing tube would be removed shortly thereafter. Fortunately, everything went fine and we rolled him into the ICU shortly after noon. David was still asleep and paralyzed from the anesthesia at first but was beginning to open his eyes a couple of hours later when I went by to visit.

His wife and teenage son were in the room. The boy seemed a little intimidated by the monitoring machinery, but McCaslin's wife stood next to the intensive care bed, holding his hand. The respirator was giving him a breath every five seconds. It was essentially doing all of his breathing. David needed to wake up enough that we could be sure he'd breathe fully on his own before we took out his breathing tube. And in order to get him from total ventilator support to total "David" support, the respiratory therapist needed to test his strength by "weaning" him off the ventilator in progressive stages.

What this means in today's practice is that his ICU nurse first has to notice he's waking up, and when she thinks he's awake enough, she'll call the respiratory therapist to come lower the ventilator rate. The nurse ordinarily is covering at least one other patient as well, and the therapist may have ten or more. Depending on whether or not there is a protocol, a doctor may also need to write an order for each ventilator change. And there may be several cycles of rate changes before everyone is comfortable that the patient is able to breathe on his own, so lots of complicated, human-dependent steps are necessary.

As it happened, I passed through the ICU again at 5 PM on the day of David McCaslin's aortic valve replacement, and he saw me walking by the room. He couldn't yell, because the breathing tube was in his mouth blocking his vocal cords, so he got my attention by hitting the side rail of his bed with his suction catheter, making a sharp rapping sound. I looked over and saw that he was alone in his room and gesturing at me; his wife had gone for tea. He was wide awake, sitting upright and pointing vehemently at the tube in his mouth. His nonverbal message was clear. He was ready to get the damn thing out, but we, the medical machinery, hadn't figured that out yet. As is often the case, the nurse and respiratory therapist were occupied with other patients, so there was no "reflexive" medical response.

The simple knee-jerk nerve circuit is probably exactly what the very first nervous systems looked like. They consisted of simple sets of neural circuits connecting distant parts of the body. In a small, primitive, brainless worm, for example, a protective reflex circuit might cause the body muscles to contract in response to and on the same side as an irritating stimulus, thereby bending the trunk away from the problem. With time, these simple nervous systems evolved, and it became useful, and evolutionarily advantageous, to develop a bundle of nerves at the front end—the feeding end—of the animal. Feeding is a critical function, and it made sense for nature to cluster sensor and effector nerves together near the mouth to make sure food got into it. That's why the brain ended up at the front rather than at the back end.

As the brain became increasingly sophisticated during evolution, reflexes became much more sophisticated. The newborn human baby, for example, has an entire suite of sophisticated reflexes designed to assist in feeding as well as in other survival functions. The *rooting reflex* helps the infant find her mother's nipple. When the infant's cheek is stroked, she'll turn her head to that side and move it around in smaller and smaller arcs until she finds the nipple with her lips, at which point the *sucking reflex* takes over.

These primitive feeding reflexes are present at birth but disappear by four months of age under normal circumstances as the growing brain takes voluntary control of the search for food. And while it would be reasonable to assume that these complicated reflex behaviors should permanently disappear after infancy, they actually only become dormant and can reemerge later in brain-damaged people. In severe Alzheimer's disease, for example, the patient can slowly regress, as if the clock were winding back, progressively losing skills like language, memories and coordination, and eventually those very primitive rooting and sucking reflexes sometimes reemerge.

Another early reflex, the *grasp*, occurs when an infant's palm is stroked. The newborn's fingers and fist close around a parent's finger, for example, in response to this stimulus. While there's nothing more heart-warming than having an infant grab your thumb, it's really only a reflex that probably evolved to keep the baby mammal clinging to his mother's once hairy back as she traveled. The *Moro reflex*, in which an infant reacts to an unexpected stimulus by extending her legs and head while flexing and grasping with her arms has the same "hanging on" function for a furry species—fortunately one that still works with a modern, clothed, mother.

There are all sorts of curious primitive reflexes that no longer have any relevance to modern living. A man's testicle pulls protectively up into the scrotum when his thigh is stroked on the same side. This is called the *cremasteric reflex*. The human heart rate slows and blood vessels constrict in the mammalian *diving reflex*. A newborn baby makes reflexive swimming movements when she's immersed in water, and when her feet are placed on a flat surface, she'll make automatic stepping movements. It's as if the newborn comes with a preprogrammed set of land and sea navigation instructions. A number of other crawling and reaching reflexes appear transiently and then disappear within the first months of a child's life.

All of these reflexes share a common set of design principles. A noxious stimulus like heat is sensed by a bodily receptor, such as the thermoreceptors in the skin. These sensor cells send a message to the central nervous system via a sensory nerve. In the spinal cord or the primitive brain, the sensing nerve interacts directly with an effector nerve which, in turn, reacts to set an evolutionarily desirable response in motion. The response may be simple, as in the knee jerk, or more complicated, as with stepping and swimming reflexes. Sneezes, coughs, salivation and blinks are all reflexive. Curiously, certain automatic facial expressions appear to be reflexive and universal, like the ones demonstrating anger and surprise that are identical in cultures around the world.

Reflexes are designed to occur very quickly—faster than the mind can think—to preserve the equilibrium of the body or to respond to a threat. So, compared to a true "thought process," reflex mechanisms are pretty simple. In fact, reflex pathways are typically so uncomplicated, albeit very elegant, that they are hard-wired so as to never interfere with or slow down conscious thought.

If our modern brains had to look after all of the things that reflexes ordinarily take care of automatically, we would never have time to smell a rose, write a poem, jump for sheer joy or get around to doing the very research it took to figure out how reflexes work. We'd be too busy just trying to coordinate all of the muscles in our legs in order to stay upright, which is the problem with modern medical care. We're all so busy trying to coordinate all of the complicated things involved in taking care of a patient that we have less and less time to think about what we're doing, and we make more and more errors. Fortunately, much of what we do in the future in medicine will eventually become much more automated and reflexive, mimicking nature's highly efficient counterparts and freeing the hands and brains of our doctors and nurses.

As a thought experiment, let's try to imagine what it would be like if you were born without the muscle spindles and reflexes responsible for the knee-jerk I described earlier, and you had to voluntarily control your legs along with the rest of the postural muscles. And just to challenge your system a little more than usual, let's pretend you've just stepped onto a moving sidewalk at an airport. Your whole body is suddenly accelerated forward, and then, because you were born without muscle spindles or reflexes, you need to *think* your way through the activities needed to stay upright in this newly precarious situation rather than letting reflexes handle it as the rest of us do.

The first thing that happens is that the balance centers in your ears send an urgent message to the brain saying, in effect, "Uh-oh, we're moving forward!" Your brain then checks around and ultimately determines that "nobody here in the brain control center ordered this movement. Let's get all hands on deck to stay upright while we figure out what the heck is going on!" The motor cortex and cerebellum are summoned to help work out a solution, and the resulting brain committee concludes, "We need to contract a lot of muscles just enough to stay erect without lurching."

After a brief sidebar, the motor cortex and cerebellum decide that this contraction will involve the calf, quadriceps, gluteal, abdominal, upper back and back of the neck muscles—the same muscles you'd use to jump or crouch with. Of course, the brain committee also told the shin, hamstring, low back and anterior neck muscles—the antagonists to the crouching muscles—to relax at the same time. This approach works fine at first but then there's a need for a big compensatory reaction, and what eventually results looks like the scarecrow when he first steps off his pole in *The Wizard of Oz*. Eventually, at the far end of the walkway, everything comes tumbling down. There is just too much conscious activity for the brain to coordinate.

Those of us who actually do have muscle spindles, unlike the guy in our thought experiment, have a much more efficient system in which the brain has delegated postural control to the reflexes that come standard with the vehicle. In a very real sense, we can actually see the human's nervous system being calibrated as our toddlers make their initial unsteady steps.

Over the first couple of days, the new walker stands up, lurches back and forth and then falls—just like the scarecrow and the guy on the people mover. But over a remarkably short period of time, too short for many parents, he's off and running, and touching, and sending everything everywhere. As he gains confidence and competence, his brain is thinking up ways to test out this delightful new capability (and vex his parents), rather than consciously controlling each and every muscle. Even a very young experienced walker can transition onto and off of a moving sidewalk with nary a lurch, because his muscle spindles, nerves and postural muscles work reflexively as a network to maintain stability without conscious thought. And his brain can take over whenever it feels necessary—like when the toddler feels it is appropriate to drop to the ground and pitch a fit.

Now, let's use the metaphor of the man on a moving sidewalk to illustrate what we do with really sick patients today and how we'll handle the same activities in the future once we've introduced medical reflex circuits into our care. Let's imagine the sudden transition from solid ground to moving surface as analogous to the transition from health to sickness, perhaps due to an overwhelming infection. I see patients like this every day in the intensive care unit, who are healthy one minute and sick as hell the next.

Our job as doctors and nurses is to look after the suddenly disrupted functions of the critically ill body, like heart rate, blood pressure, breathing, and kidney and—most importantly—brain function. The body ordinarily does this reflexively, but sickness throws those reflexes out of whack, and we end up trying to correct those functions with medicines, IV fluids, respirators, diuretics and the like. The medical result is often very much like the lurching of the scarecrow or the toddler—uncoordinated and fitful. The healthy body ordinarily does this really well.

For example, if a critically ill patient's blood pressure begins to drop, an alarm rings, summoning a nurse; the nurse determines that the alarm is real and calls a doctor; the doctor thinks and comes up with a treatment; the treatment is ordered; and then the nurse administers it. To be sure, this is all done speedily in an ICU, but the whole process is *much* slower than the body's reflex reaction is. In the future, however, the medical response will be much more automated and more like a reflex.

The patient will still lie surrounded by similar medicine pumps and machines, but the machines of the future will be a little bit smarter than the current ones. And we'll use a network of medical sensors equivalent to the muscle spindle that will automatically sense sudden changes in heart rate, blood pressure, breathing and kidney function. These sensors will be connected by wires, like nerves, or wirelessly to the equipment around the patient, and we'll let the machines respond to any disturbance with automatic corrective action, just like your postural muscles respond instantly and automatically when you step on a moving sidewalk.

As with humans, the brain—be it the doctor's or the nurse's—can always override the automatic network, just as a pilot can override an autopilot. This same automated approach is already being used to control the administration of some medications in research settings. The blood sugar of diabetics is sensed continuously and the values used to control the automatic administration of insulin in what's called a closed-loop system and amounts to an artificial pancreas.

The range and variety of medical devices designed to measure things about a patient is mind numbing. The medical device manufacturing industry has exploded over the past 50 years. In my father's era, the stethoscope, blood pressure cuff and a finger on the pulse sufficed for most routine examinations. Today's "executive physical" involves a comprehensive examination and a battery of analyses including blood tests for diabetes, anemia, thyroid, liver and kidney disease; a lipid panel to assess cardiac and stroke risk factors; a stool test to check for gastrointestinal bleeding, an electrocardiogram, a chest x-ray for heart size, pulmonary function testing, an audiogram for signs of hearing loss and an eye exam; colon cancer screening, skin cancer screening; prostate screening in men and a mammogram, pap smear and bone-density study for women. Some even include a total body "screening" CT scan. The sicker the patient, the greater the degree of monitoring and data collection. Patients in the operating room and intensive care unit are surrounded by monitoring devices, and state-of-the-art interventional radiology and cardiology laboratories are like spaceships.

Medicine is saturated with sensors. We collect more information than we know what to do with today. In our ICU for example, the nurse transcribes into the medical record only a tiny fraction of the heart rate, blood pressure and other data we measure continuously with sensors. And while we're *sensor* rich, our *responses* are still very manual. There's very little in the way of automated, reflexive medical care, but there's every reason to move in that direction.

You'd think that if we can make autopilots that we trust to fly jets full of people, we could make a ventilator capable of weaning itself by sensing when a patient like David McCaslin is ready to breathe on his own. I actually asked a ventilator manufacturer about this recently, and he told me the capability is actually *already* built into the microcircuitry of the machine but that we don't use it because the medical industry is just too conservative to routinely turn medical functions over to machines—that is, to allow machines to become autonomous doctors. We haven't evolved that far yet, he seemed to suggest.

In fact, we routinely insert smart pacemaker/defibrillators, called *automatic implanted cardioverter defibrillators* or AICDs, into patients every day. These are essentially autonomous cardiologists, fully trained to diagnose a wide range of heart rhythm abnormalities and empowered to automatically defibrillate the heart if appropriate. Letting a microchip deliver a jolt of electricity into the center of the heart when it's fibrillating is directly analogous to letting an airline autopilot apply full power and dive in response to a stall. It's also like the human body's own emergency fight-or-flight reflex, in which adrenaline is pumped into the circulation to put all systems on full "go" mode. In each instance, an emergency response is designed to occur extremely quickly and at a subconscious level.

As medicine continues to evolve, automatic, autonomous, or closed-loop sensor-controlled loops—reflexes—will become common. A smart, self-weaning ventilator will allow nurses and respiratory therapists to care for more patients with greater safety and efficiency. Smart insulin pumps will improve blood sugar control and decrease the need for micromanagement by the diabetic patient. In the near future, your smartphone may well tell you that you've been sitting on your duff all day and to get moving, or, perhaps, that your heart rate went too high on that last flight of steps—maybe even that you need to see a doctor immediately because your heart's in trouble.

Your home-health network will probably monitor your weight; blood pressure; perhaps even the composition of your breath, urine or stool; and give you information about how to adjust your diet or medications. The common denominator for all of these mechanisms is that there is no human doctor or nurse in the loop. They happen below the level of traditional medical consciousness, like a reflex. In the same way that evolution favored reflex responses, it will eventually favor medical interventions that can occur automatically, freeing high-level costly assets like the doctor and the nurse for more complicated tasks.

The brain is extremely efficient at delegating work. We've all had the sensation of finding ourselves in the midst of a complicated activity like walking or swimming and realizing that our minds are "elsewhere." You're walking just fine, but your brain went on to other things after having delegated a routine function to some walking or swimming subroutine. Medicine doesn't do this very well today, but it will. Much of what we now do manually will soon become standardized and automatic.

David McCaslin will be weaned from the ventilator automatically by a weaning subroutine built in to the machine, which frees the brains and hands of the doctor, respiratory therapist and nurse. They will only need to get involved when something deviates from the routine. From McCaslin's standpoint, this is a much more satisfactory approach than having to bang on the side rails to get my attention. And, assuming the subroutine is written properly, it may even be safer. Just as it's usually safer not to think too much about walking, it's sometimes safer to let machines perform the same proven process over and over, only calling in a human for exceptions or problems.

The health-care system is crying to be automated and standardized. Many practices that doctors and nurses currently *think* their way through, often way too deliberately, are slowly becoming standardized and reflexive already. To give you an example of what I mean, when I was a resident, a patient who developed a new fever with low blood pressure used to go through an extensive evaluation while the doctor tried to decide which antibiotics were appropriate.

We'd perform an x-ray of the chest and collect samples of sputum, urine, blood and sometimes spinal fluid; depending on the results, a specific set of antibacterial or antifungal drugs would be initiated. Five patients with the exact same findings in this workup might end up on five different drug regimens, and the average time to beginning treatment might well be hours. During these hours, the patient isn't getting *any* antibiotics at all. All of the *thinking* was getting in the way of *action*. Today we do things differently and act more reflexively. When today's patient develops a fever and low blood pressure in our hospital or emergency room, as well as at many other hospitals around the country, the *sepsis protocol* for overwhelming infections is initiated. Like a reflex, the sepsis protocol is a highly standardized set of actions initiated automatically in response to a problem. Just as the knee jerks when the patella is struck, we perform a standard set of lab measurements, blood analyses, treatments to restore blood pressure and, most importantly, start a standard set of broad-spectrum antibiotics as quickly as possible. The antibiotics are part of the sepsis *bundle*. The development of this sepsis protocol has saved lives. More and more standardized routines like this are being developed for patient care as we come to better understand best practices for other diseases like this one for bad infections.

The evolutionarily successful doctor of the future may well only step in when his patient strays significantly off a course that is largely managed by protocol. Many of my medical colleagues who have always done things their own way will protest that these protocols are bad and that every patient is *different,* just as tailors of a different era must have protested that every man has a unique and different shape and that the bespoke suit was the only kind to wear. Standardized sizes and sewing patterns came into being during the Civil War, when it became necessary to churn out uniforms. At the beginning of the war, uniforms were made by government contractors working from their homes, but factories took over as demand grew. It became apparent that men clustered into predictable sets of measurements, which led to the development of standard sizes and thence to the evolution of ready-made clothing. In reality, a lot of the variation in modern medical care is a matter of style rather than proven substance. Patients can be grouped into standard sets, and we can provide treatments at much lower expense and often more safely by using more of the mass-production, templated approaches espoused by Henry Kaiser and Sidney Garfield.

Reflexes developed as a solution to the growing complexity of the evolving animal. Simple animals had simple reflexes. More complicated animals, like the human, have a varied and extensive suite of reflexes. A reflex is the nervous system's protocol or program for dealing with a recurring problem. Dust flies into the eye and we blink and tear; up the nose, we sneeze and our nose runs; into the lungs, we cough and make secretions. These are complicated, organized, reproducible and automatic responses to problems the body knows about. Many medical problems are equally familiar and well understood by the medical profession, and we need to evolve the same sorts of standardized responses for asthma, diabetes, hypertension and pneumonia to replace the one-off, bespoke solutions we too often adopt today.

Doctors and nurses of the future will spend more of their time handling those patients who *deviate* from the routine or predictable, and much less in doing mundane, easily automated tasks. They'll act like the modern brain does, taking on complicated tasks that are beyond the scope of a reflex. For example, a telemedical intensive care specialist can look after over a hundred patients in several ICUs simultaneously with the assistance of automated smart alarms that act like muscle spindle sensors and notify him only when something is wrong with a patient's vital signs. He doesn't need to spend time seeking important information; it is brought to him, dramatically increasing his efficiency. Anesthesiologists may well work similarly in the future, covering several operating rooms at the same time from a control center. And this same model can be extended to home care.

Elderly, recently hospitalized or chronically ill patients are already beginning to have medical equipment installed in their homes and networked from their local computer and thereby to the internet. These devices sense the patient just like a muscle spindle: assessing for blood pressure, blood sugar, weight or heart rate abnormalities. When the system senses a problem, perhaps an alarmingly high blood pressure or heart rate, it can make some immediate recommendations to the patient and simultaneously send an alarm through the network to a command center staffed by nurses and doctors. Depending on the nature of the problem, these providers may send help immediately, via an ambulance, or reach out to the patient over an audiovisual link using a tool like Cisco's HealthPresence telemedicine tool designed to network doctors and patients in a nearly immersive environment.

As medical equipment becomes increasingly electronic and networked, we are essentially developing a nervous system extending all the way and continuously from the doctor and nurse to the patient, who may be walking around with a sophisticated medical brain in a holster clipped to his belt. Cheap, disposable, muscle-spindle-like sensors will be embedded in our clothes, sneakers, bandages and jewelry. In fact, the Chilean miners who spent more than two months trapped underground in a 2010 mine accident wore sensors that could continuously measure blood pressure, blood oxygen saturation, heart rate, respiratory rate and posture—to determine whether or not the wearer had fallen—and wirelessly transmit it to cell phones that were carried by each. These smartphones were delivered to the miners through a small relief hole that was successfully drilled 2,300 feet through the earth's crust to reach them. As cell phones and home-based devices begin to generate medical information from non-hospitalized individuals, the volume of resulting information will be too overwhelming for any human to evaluate, and we will be forced to rely on automated, smart solutions to sort the wheat from the chaff. Computers like IBM's Jeopardy champion, Watson, will live in the middle of the medical internet, automatically predigesting medical data for action by human providers.

Health care is poised for dramatic change, and we're barreling toward an era of really smart medicine.

CHAPTER 12

DOCTORS IN FLIGHT

In retrospect, they all agreed that the thing that tripped up Maurice Gutierrez's doctor was the part about the room spinning. Maurice had called Dr. O'Neal earlier to say that he felt sick to his stomach and had a headache, and that every time he stood up, he felt dizzy. So the doctor's first thought was to prescribe a motion-sickness pill. Gutierrez had actually had a headache for almost a week now, but the dizziness, which Dr. O'Neal called *vertigo,* had come on suddenly.

Gutierrez's wife found a 24-hour pharmacy and picked up some Dramamine at O'Neal's recommendation, but it hadn't done anything other than to make him feel groggier with no relief for the headache. But the whole situation changed alarmingly when his right arm and leg started to tingle and go numb. Worse yet, he also found he was having trouble explaining what was going on to his increasingly alarmed wife; he couldn't seem to find the words, or else garbled them. She called Dr. O'Neal back, and he told her to take her husband to the hospital *immediately.*

By the time they arrived at the emergency room of their small local hospital, Maurice was no longer able to move his right side and had to be helped out of the car by an orderly into the wheelchair. The alert triage nurse recognized what might be going on and had him seen immediately by the doctor despite the fact that the waiting room was full of patients who had been there much longer. The emergency medical doctor's provisional diagnosis was "possible CVA," which is shorthand for *cerebrovascular accident.* This really means that he suspected something had gone very wrong with the blood supply to Maurice's brain, a very reasonable presumption. The doctor could have been even more specific, given the fact that the left half of the human brain controls the right half of the body and the major speech centers are also typically located on the left. He could have written "possible L hemispheric CVA." This was almost certainly a big, left-brain stroke.

We've made tremendous advances recently in our understanding of what happens in the brain during a stroke, how long it takes between the onset of symptoms and irreversible damage, and how to handle problems like clots for which we actually have treatments that work, and thereby save the brain, if they're administered soon enough. It wasn't long ago that a patient like Maurice would come into an ER with an evolving stroke, and we doctors would stand by helplessly, knowing that the resulting paralysis and speech problems would probably be permanent and devastating. Today, however, we have drugs that can dissolve clots and restore blood flow. The only problem is that strokes have two major causes, and while clot-busting treatment can save the life of some patients, it can kill others—the ones with bleeding rather than clot. Stroke experts have developed a standard approach designed to quickly tell them what is going on, how bad it is and whether or not to treat with clot drugs. There are three major elements.

The first is *time*. Because stroke patients may be unconscious or unable to determine the exact time of onset of their symptoms, neurologists use the term "last seen well" as a guide to how long a patient's brain may have been deprived of blood flow. The second element involves the determination of a patient's stroke *score*. Two common scoring systems are the American National Institutes of Health Stroke Scale and the Canadian Neurologic Score. The systems provide a very objective score of brain damage by checking level of consciousness, visual findings, facial muscles, arms, legs, balance, sensation and language. This test is designed to be administered quickly so that the patient can then be whisked off to a CT scanner for the third test, to determine whether or not there is bleeding in the brain, which would eliminate the patient as a candidate for clot-busting treatment.

As soon as the scan is complete, the stroke score is reassessed. If the value either is improving or has dropped too low, the risks of clot busting outweigh the potential benefits of the treatment, so it is not started. But if the neurological symptoms haven't improved, and the CT scan shows no hemorrhage, treatment is started immediately. The goal is to treat within a three-hour window of the onset of symptoms; to push this, stroke care advocates have come up with a campaign based on the compelling phrase "Time is Brain." Incidentally, this whole protocol is another example of reflexive, automatic, "best-practice" routines, like the ones I described in the previous chapter, that are becoming prevalent in medical care.

Maurice was seen promptly, and his CT scan was completed within 45 minutes of his arrival. But things broke down thereafter because there wasn't a radiologist on site, so, unfortunately, his scan wasn't read for an hour and a half. During this waiting period, which he spent in the emergency room, his speech difficulties worsened. His wife was terrified because he was no longer able to say anything that made sense, but he was clearly trying to communicate *something* with urgency. The frustration and fear were written all over his face.

When the scan was finally read, it showed no abnormalities, which is often the case in the first hours after an embolic stroke. The word *embolism* actually derives from a Greek word meaning a "plug," and a clot that plugs up a major cerebral artery can cause symptoms like Maurice's, suggesting that a large portion of brain tissue is not getting blood flow and is about to suffer irreparable damage. In fact, within less than 24 hours, if left untreated, the scan of a patient with a big stroke will eventually show swelling and abnormalities in the gray and white matter of the brain.

This is very much like what happens with a bruise on the skin. One of the body's universal responses to injury is swelling, as blood vessels in the region become leaky, allowing white cells to move into the injured tissue. Months and years later, a stroke patient's scan will show a hole in the brain where the normal brain tissue used to be. Sadly, this is what would eventually happen to Maurice Gutierrez, because by the time his scan was read, he was already outside the safe time window for clot-busting treatment. A portion of his brain had died. For Maurice, indeed, Time was Brain—lost brain, in this case.

Like the emergency room the Gutierrezes went to, the typical emergency center is not yet prepared to provide round-the-clock stroke diagnosis and treatment, which is unfortunate, because stroke and heart attack are two of the most common and most devastating complications of the Western lifestyle. The American Stroke Association has actually defined recommendations for the establishment of Stroke Systems of Care, designed to streamline and coordinate the entire continuum of stroke management—from prevention to rehabilitation—and across all of the facilities involved in that continuum.

The Brain Attack Coalition is centered at the U.S. National Institute of Neurological Diseases and Stroke and coordinates the efforts of neurologists, neurosurgeons, neurological nurses, emergency medical doctors and paramedics in defining best-practice protocols. Their checklist for communities includes items like: (1) Does the community's hospital have a stroke team that can evaluate a patient within 15 minutes of arrival? (2) Are the community's emergency medical systems designed to transport suspected stroke patients to the hospital as rapidly as possible? (3) Is there a neurosurgeon available around the clock? and (4) Can the hospital perform *and interpret* a CT scan within 45 minutes of a suspected stroke patient's admission? This fourth element is, of course, where things went wrong for Maurice. To be fair, most areas of the United States and the rest of world lack coordinated stroke care, and the resources to develop and maintain stroke centers are considerable because they require immediate, round-the-clock access to specialists like stroke specialists and neuroradiologists.

Strokes are an example of acute medical problems that occur infrequently enough in any one area that it makes sense to develop systems to either rapidly move expert care to the patient (like emergency helicopters sometimes bring nurses, paramedics and doctors to accident scenes) or move the patient to a specialized facility (as by helicopter to a trauma center). The flight capabilities of helicopters have revolutionized trauma care, and medical helicopters have been conscripted in some areas to facilitate the transport of patients to stroke centers. The state of Ohio has taken flight one giant, technologically sophisticated step further, in the design of its comprehensive Heart Disease and Stroke Prevention Plan.

Stroke treatment is "virtually" flown to underserved and remote rural hospitals in Ohio through a system of stroke telemedicine networks. These small hospitals have an always-on telemedical connection to the stroke center, and the minute a patient like Maurice arrives, a stroke specialist—a neurologist—at a remote, core hospital is engaged in his care. The mechanics of this arrangement are pretty simple. The stroke specialist sits in front of a camera- and microphone-enabled computer at one end, and a typically mobile unit is wheeled into the patient's room. A video screen on the mobile unit displays the doctor's face to the patient, while a camera on the unit allows the doctor to see the patient. Two-way audio completes the connection so that the stroke neurologist can examine the patient with the assistance of a nurse or family member, asking appropriate questions and going through a physical examination.

Using the telemedical link, the stroke specialist can establish when the patient was last seen well, perform the required initial stroke scale testing, read the CT scan and then complete the follow-up stroke scale. The neurologist is able to perform all of these critical functions remotely—so he can cover lots of facilities simultaneously from one geographic location—and then make the decision as to whether treatment with a clot-busting drug is appropriate. The goal of the Ohio Department of Health is to ensure that *all* of its residents have access to immediate stroke care throughout the state and to thereby prevent whenever possible what ultimately happened to Maurice Gutierrez, with its human and long-term financial costs. This obviously has benefits for the individual patient and also makes economic sense for a state that will bear a significant portion of the costs of any consequent long-term disability a patient may sustain after a stroke.

Like sight, flight represented an enormous evolutionary advantage for species that developed the capability. There are several hypotheses as to why flight evolved in the first place, one or more of which may be true. Some evolutionary scientists believe that primitive flight developed as an escape mechanism while others feel it was a mechanism for catching elusive prey; still others think that arms became wings to free up the hind legs as weapons.

Two other theories of flight's roots are directly relevant to the way medicine will evolve in the future. Wings may actually have evolved to permit *rapid movement from one place to another* or to allow a species to *gain access to an unoccupied ecological niche*. It is by analogy to these ecological drivers that we can compare telemedicine, or medicine from afar, to flight. Absent telemedical links, there would be no stroke centers in rural Ohio, and these portions of the state therefore represent unoccupied niches for stroke doctors. Similar opportunities exist all over the world, representing an enormous evolutionary prospect for flight-capable, telemedical practitioners. Telemedicine actually represents an easy way to address the huge inequities in medical care between the underserved and the, arguably, overserved populations of the world.

I recently had a chance to meet with the doctors and administrators of a small but very good hospital along the coast of Maine, the Mount Desert

Island (MDI) Hospital. This hospital serves several distinct patient populations with discrete needs. In the summer, hoards of transient summer vacationers flood the area, bringing with them a particular but predictable set of problems. There are, for example, the chest, muscle and joint pains of the suddenly hyperactive desk jockey up for a week of fun, hiking and climbing in Acadia National Park. The town of Bar Harbor also has its share of drunks and drug overdoses, sunburns and barnacle injuries. There are also the very serious traumatic injuries that occur when a human falls from almost any height onto Maine's adamantine granite, and the park provides many opportunities for harm, including excursions like a cliff hike along "The Precipice," an exposed 1,000-foot climb on the east face of Champlain Mountain.

MDI Hospital also has a second population of patients with its year-round residents. These are the tough people who have chosen to live in Maine all through its four seasons: the brief summers, the lovely "shoulder seasons" in the spring and fall, and its tough, cold, hard winters. Many of these make the bulk of their income during the summer when the area is flush with tourist money and then must husband their resources through the winter. Some farm. There are fishermen, lobstermen, loggers and all manner of others who work with their hands. They have the same medical issues the rest of us deal with, but they're less likely to seek medical help until forced to, by pain or disability—a pattern of medical stoicism that is much less common in other, medically lush parts of the country. And some of these folks live on one of the more than 1,000 islands along Maine's coast. For them, a trip to the doctor involves at least two boat voyages, there and back again. Mental illness, in the form of depression or substance abuse, is common, particularly during the isolation of winter, when many people are shut in for long periods of time.

There is also a third group of patients who use and care about this little hospital; while small in number, this group has a significant impact on the way the hospital sees its mission. Like other spectacular parts of the world, Maine's coast attracts a transient population of people of substantial means who come to the area during a particular season—in Maine, it's the summer—but remain invested in its welfare throughout the year. John D. Rockefeller is the perfect example of an extremely wealthy, philanthropically oriented visitor to this part of Maine. He was an avid horseman and spearheaded the development of the carriage roads and vistas of Acadia's park. Today's philanthropists are carrying on his spirit by ensuring that the area is served with advanced medical care. These modern Maine patrons are developing a program to "fly" tertiary care to the MDI hospital via telemedical links, rather than flying out its patients.

MDI Hospital already uses telemedical links to connect its own clinicians based in the small emergency room with medical providers located or rounding on the tiny Big and Little Moose, Heron and Bald Porcupine Islands, which are scattered offshore around the much bigger Mount Desert Island. But MDI's benefactors would also like to connect its doctors with tertiary care experts, like a neurologist, cardiologist, psychiatrist or even a dermatologist, when their specific services are required.

Let's say, for example, that Maurice Gutierrez had arrived at the MDI emergency room with his evolving neurological symptoms. MDI is not currently a stroke center but, with a telemedical link to a tertiary center, it could become one in an instant. Similarly, MDI is too small to have a full-time intensive care specialist, much less round-the-clock coverage by an intensive care team; the ICU has only three beds. But, with the assistance of telemedicine, an intensive care team at a tertiary care center could look after MDI's patients as well as those of several other small hospitals around the country, simultaneously and economically.

Wings evolved over a period of hundreds of millions of years, and, while seemingly modern, telemedicine, too, has ancient roots. The first telemedical application actually dates back to the first years of the twentieth century, when doctors attempted to transmit the sounds of the heart and breathing over telephone lines to remote colleagues. Radio waves were later used to connect shore-based physicians with ships in the 1920s. Telepsychiatry debuted in the 1950s over closed-circuit television. And satellites were used to link paramedics in Alaskan and Canadian villages with higher level medical facilities in the 1970s. While these first historical telemedical efforts were fraught with technical problems, they are analogous to the enthusiastic first leaps of those adventurous dinosaurs that ultimately became the ancestors of today's rich and diverse class of birds.

When my father began his residency in the 1950s, he served for several years as a house officer and was essentially geographically bound to the grounds of the hospital like some fossorial, burrow-dwelling animal. His role was to be readily physically available in a very circumscribed location whenever needed. As we saw in an earlier chapter, the evolution of communication devices has given physicians increased freedom and range, while simultaneously giving patients more immediate access to the services of mobile experts. By the time I entered my own residency in the 1980s, we carried beepers that, for certain rotations, gave us the freedom to dart about relatively freely at some distance from our "burrow," as long as we remained within the radio range of the beeper and were able to get to a phone within a relatively short period of time. I would tailor my jogging routes, for example, to remain within striking distance of a pay telephone, and I always carried a quarter.

By the time I became a junior faculty member in the early 1990s, the first brick-sized cell phones had become available. Although it wasn't ideal, one could jog carrying one of these heavy two-way communication devices along less well-trodden pathways, as long as there was cell coverage. The additional freedom permitted by the cell phone permitted longer distance roaming because I no longer need to remain within reach of a phone booth. By the year 2000, I could confidently handle some of my responsibilities by cell phone from anywhere in the country. As cell phones became smaller and cheaper, at the same time that cell coverage became relatively ubiquitous, we physicians acquired the freedom to fly *really* far from our burrows.

We could now practice medicine from a distance, although admittedly with a limited set of tools—just conversations. But, as with wings, the tools and capabilities continue to evolve rapidly, and doctors in the future will be able to practice very effectively from a great distance. As we'll see, the cell phone has already become a primary medical tool in parts of the third world, linking doctors with primary providers in rural Africa, for example, or emergency medical workers from disaster-ravaged Haiti to tertiary medical centers in the United States.

The American Telemedical Association (ATA) defines telemedicine as "the use of medical information exchanged from one site to another via electronic communications to improve patients' health status."[1] This definition encompasses several different flavors of medical interactions.

Specialist referral services occur when an expert in a given field assists a general practitioner in rendering a diagnosis using live or previously captured data, such as x-rays or pictures of a skin lesion. A specialist radiologist who reads an x-ray from a remote location is providing this kind of telemedicine.

Telemedical patient consultations involve a direct link between a remote physician and a patient. Some unscrupulous, profit-minded physicians were quick to recognize the utility of the internet as a mechanism for extending their reach into previously untapped ecological niches. They quickly set up what were, in effect, pharmaceutical storefronts in the early days of network proliferation and interacted with the "patient" through questionnaires, prescribing highly sought-after drugs like Viagra and anabolic steroids for a fee.

Remote patient monitoring systems use devices to capture medical data from patients and feed it to physicians or nurses, often after some computerized predigestion through which problematic trends are identified and highlighted.

The telemedicine association also describes delivery mechanisms, ranging from networked programs linking hospitals over dedicated, high-speed lines, to point-to-point connections between hospitals and affiliated clinics. Networks also link homebound patients to providers for health maintenance and cardiac, pulmonary and fetal monitoring. Web-based portals are useful for certain kinds of more educationally oriented communications between providers and patients.

The ATA's distinctions within telemedicine are useful in categorizing the ways in which doctors can assist remote colleagues in doing their jobs or can care for patients at a distance, but medicine is quickly taking flight through ad hoc, innovative applications of available technologies that are changing so rapidly as to defy our ability to capture what's happening in any static picture.

I recently participated in a national meeting on telemedicine and saw a lecture given by Colonel Ron K. Poropatich, a physician who has been a pioneer in military telemedicine. At the time, he was the deputy director of the U.S. Army's Telemedicine and Advanced Technology Research Center at Fort Detrick, Maryland. The scope of TATRC's initiatives is breathtaking and includes e-health, the "digital warrior," medicine in austere environments, integrative medicine and the "hospital of the future."

At the meeting, Ron showed a video clip of a dramatic example of ad hoc telemedicine that ultimately saved a gravely injured soldier's life. Head injuries became alarmingly common during the Iraq and Afghanistan wars, due to both high-velocity rifle rounds and improvised explosive devices. During the more intensive phases of these wars, it was not unusual for injured soldiers to be evacuated from a battle site to a forward operating base, such as the one in Mosul, where a surgical team was positioned to provide immediate medical care.

The job of the surgical teams at forward bases is to stabilize and save the lives of soldiers: sew up bleeding vessels, amputate mangled extremities or divert spilled bowel contents into colostomy bags to prevent infection of the abdominal cavity. The definitive care for these injuries typically occurs later, at more sophisticated hospitals well behind the lines or in another country.

The required skill set for frontline army surgeons does not include cardiac or neurosurgical expertise, although some of the doctors who end up at these bases *are* cardiac surgeons, like Major Sloane Guy. Guy completed his general surgical training in the United States and went on to become a cardiac surgeon while still an active member of the military. During a tour in Afghanistan, and based on his experiences in advanced centers in the United States, he recognized that there was a pressing opportunity for what might be called *emergency teleproctoring*: a specialist physician in one discipline could guide another through an operation he hadn't previously performed, and do so from almost any distance using audiovisual links.

Working with military and industrial research organizations, Dr. Guy and Dr. Poropatich from TATRC designed an ad hoc system whereby a stateside specialist surgeon could walk and talk a frontline surgeon through a neurosurgical procedure, for example, that the latter had never before seen much less done. Guy actually used this system during a tour in Mosul, Iraq. Wearing a head-mounted camera and a Bluetooth cell-phone earpiece, he was able to operate and simultaneously stream live images to a colleague eight time zones away while the two were in continuous two-way voice communication. The U.S.-based physician could draw virtual chalk on a monitor visible to Guy in Mosul, just like a network football analyst, to show where to cut or sew. This two-way system was designed to allow a surgeon like Guy, who was trained to operate on *hearts,* to perform the stabilizing measures necessary to save the life of a five-year-old with a *head* injury or a soldier with a ruptured bladder. This same capability would have been very helpful to some of the medical teams in Haiti after the devastating January 2010 earthquake, but they made do with even lower-tech tools.

A typical Haitian-relief team consisted of anesthesiologists, surgeons and nurses whose training had been in areas like general, orthopedic and trauma surgery. There wasn't any obvious reason to include a neurosurgeon on the team because most of the initial surgical work during this disaster involved the management of broken or crushed arms and legs. But one day a young kid showed up with his mother; the boy obviously had a skull fracture; there was a huge bruise and a dent where his head had hit a rock.

He was the only child left in the family; the father and the rest of the children had been crushed in their house when it fell during the quake. Tragically, the boy's injury actually happened a full week *after* the earthquake when he fell off of his bicycle while carrying water from a well back to his mother. When he arrived at the clinic, the child was unconscious, and the medical team was concerned that there was bleeding around the brain. They felt compelled to do something, but none of them had ever operated on a head injury.

This medical team was based at a hospital that had sustained no real damage, miles away from the earthquake epicenter. It was possible to get an emergency x-ray, but the CT scanner that might have told them whether or not there was blood in the skull, and where, didn't exist here. There was, however, a working cell connection, so the team sent a cell-phone picture of the skull film showing the location of the fracture back to a neurosurgeon at their home hospital in Philadelphia. After reviewing the film, the neurosurgeon recommended a simple, relatively low-risk procedure with the potential for a high reward. *Burr hole craniotomy* refers to an operation in which a small hole is drilled in the skull, and a sterile drain is inserted through the hole and attached to suction.

If there is blood compressing and further damaging the brain, it can be drained continuously via this method; if there isn't, there's very little to be lost. The neurosurgeon told the Haitian team where to drill the burr hole based on the x-ray he'd received on his cell-phone screen. They inserted the drain under local anesthesia and were, in fact, able to suck out a significant amount of blood. The boy, Jean Jacques, woke up several hours later.

For better or for worse, we're moving to an era of "always on" medical care, and we're going to see the evolution of a class of doctors who practice their profession from a distance. Radiologists and dermatologists already do, and the tools to practice critical care, neurology, psychiatry and even medical care in the home via telemedicine are evolving rapidly. Just as the capacity to fly provided the evolving class of birds with access to new ecological niches as they branched away from the dinosaurs and provided the ability to move rapidly from one location to another, telemedical doctors will be able to bring their expertise to new parts of the country and the world and increase the geographic range of their practice almost infinitely.

The U.S. National Institute of Mental Health published a study at the end of 2009 evaluating the incidence of mental disorders among adolescents ages 8 to 15; it perfectly illustrates the parallels between the evolutionary opportunities offered by flight and telemedicine. Based on a sample of thousands of youth, the institute found that every tenth child met criteria for one or more mental disorders, including attention-deficit hyperactivity disorder (ADHD), depression, "conduct" disorder, anxiety or an eating disorder.

More boys had ADHD than girls, and more girls suffered from depression and eating disorders. ADHD was more common in lower socioeconomic groups, as were mental problems in general, while higher socioeconomic children were more likely to suffer from anxiety syndromes like panic disorder. Autism, bipolar and borderline personality disorders, schizophrenia and suicide affect children as well as adults. All of these diseases have both short-term and lifelong consequences; early recognition and treatment can improve lives immeasurably or save them. Unfortunately, there aren't enough doctors who know how to manage these problems to go around.

Although the services of an adolescent psychiatrist are readily available in some parts of the country, they're not in others. In fact, the discrepancy between the number of psychiatrists per 100,000 youth from state to state is dramatic. The District of Columbia is the leader with 42 per 100,000; Massachusetts, Connecticut and Maryland have about 20 per 100,000; and big empty states like Alaska, Nevada and Wyoming have only about 3 qualified psychiatrists for every 100,000 youth—even though every tenth kid might benefit from their services.

Telepsychiatry is a "poster child" model for telemedical care. First of all, it has been proven to work. And, it's a win-win proposition for both doctors *and* patients. Imagine all those poor shrinks in DC elbowing each other out of the way to get a piece of the action in Washington's overcrowded ecosystem, while across the country there are thousands of underserved kids. Every country in the world has similar problems with regional mismatches between supply and demand: too many doctors in desirable locations and too few for most of the population. But more importantly, the patients telemedically served can stay in their homes or travel only a short distance for their care.

By eliminating the need for the doctor to be within easy driving distance of the patient, everyone wins. The first pioneer telepsychiatry practices are already appearing on the web. One site advertises therapy "by telephone or webcam, in the convenience and privacy of home." As this entrepreneurial psychiatrist puts it, "I use either the telephone or a phone and webcam, with or without a chat service. My most popular arrangement is to use Skype with a webcam; after a few minutes it feels as if we are in the room together! I do not prescribe strong controlled substances by telepsychiatry for obvious reasons."

This particular psychiatrist has both a physical and a virtual telemedical practice. He spends some of his time practicing on the ground and some in an on-air practice. Similarly, neurologists who practice telestroke care, the ones who might have treated Maurice Gutierrez before the brain damage became permanent, typically practice both at the bedside and over the airwaves. Both the stateside surgeon who mentored Dr. Sloane Guy through unfamiliar operations in Afghanistan and Iraq, and Guy himself operate on very real patients every day, but their novel use of telemedical techniques shows another way in which even surgery is leaping into the air and gives us a peek at how medicine may be practiced in the future. Some of today's radiologists practice exclusively online from their homes. All of the equipment they need to read films is located in their home offices, and they never have to wear a white coat to work; they could, for all intents and purposes, be practicing from another planet.

As the tools with which we interface to the internet become more robust, medical practice will continue to evolve quickly. Videoconferencing over cell phones will soon become commonplace. Wearable gesture interfaces (such as the SixthSense device designed by Pranav Mistry from the Massachusetts Institute of Technology's Media Lab) combine sensors, a camera and a projector; they permit the wearer to transition almost transparently from the real to the digital world. These new technologies will eventually blur the distinction between the kinds of medicine that can be practiced effectively using telemedical wings and those that require the physical presence of a physician. Mobile health is currently in its nascence, but the forces supporting its evolution, ranging from governments and corporations to patient advocates and providers, make its evolution inevitable.

CHAPTER 13

MEDICAL AVATARS

On a typical weekend night, there are at least 20 to 30 people in our emergency room waiting area, sitting in various degrees of comfort and sobriety on hard plastic chairs—the kind from which blood and other bodily liquids can be readily wiped. I pass through this area rarely, typically after a late case in the operating room and at a time when our hospital security staff are channeling traffic through a limited number of doors.

I'm usually in scrubs when I leave at these hours and therefore very clearly a medical professional of some sort, and waiting people stare hungrily at me when I pass, hoping I'm coming to talk to them. Many have been sitting for hours on those plastic seats, which are uncomfortable under the best of circumstances but all the more so when one's ill and would prefer to be in bed.

There are lots of reasons people come to emergency rooms in the middle of the night. The most common complaint for men is chest pain, while for women it's stomach pain or abdominal cramps. And while men and women have back pain in about the same proportion, men are much more likely to have cuts and car accidents while women describe nausea and cough symptoms.

One of the most critical jobs in an ER is the determination of which patients need to be seen first. An ER is not like a bank or a ticket office, where it's first come, first served. The rules of engagement for an ER are the same as those of a newspaper: "If it bleeds, it leads." The sickest patients jump, as they should, to the head of the queue, and the person making the prioritization determination is typically the triage nurse. It's the triage nurse's job to sort patients into categories.

While many countries use different systems, their triage systems all have some equivalent to a "priority 1," where the patient is unconscious, unresponsive or has other life threatening injuries—like the not-unheard-of situation in which someone walks into triage with lots of stab wounds. The patients who wait longest in ERs are at the other end of the spectrum, and these "priority 5" patients often have some minor complaint, like a sore throat.

Triage categories don't always map directly or accurately onto how sick a patient really is, of course. I've taken care of unconscious, priority-1 patients who turned out to be just drunk, as well as drunks who also had bleeding into their brains. I've also seen patients with what they described as a sore throat, when the throat pain actually turned out to be the clue to an evolving heart attack. However subjective it may sometimes turn out to be, triage is an essential function.

Today's ERs are invariably overtaxed, and hospitals have done what they can to distract the waiters. Television is a near-universal panacea. The Children's Hospital of Philadelphia has cartoons and movies on television, game consoles and a large kinetic sculpture with balls that funnel through a complicated obstacle course making loud, but distracting, sounds as they bounce off things and one another.

There was actually a tropical fish tank in our own ER at one point, but legend (perhaps urban) has it that it shattered during an altercation among several frisky "patients," and some said that gunplay was involved. A metal detector appeared at the door to the waiting room around this same period.

Performed efficiently, triage can funnel hundreds of patients safely through a busy city ER on a single night. On the other hand, one error can be fatal. Joaquin Rivera was a well-known, Philadelphia-based, Puerto Rican high-school counselor and musician.[1] A community activist and the father of three, he was 63 years old on the night he went to a nearby hospital at 10:45 PM with pain in his left chest, arm and belly—those all-too-common complaints for men. Rivera had walked alone to the hospital from his home four blocks away and was told by the triage nurse to sit in the waiting area. But he wasn't alone there, as security camera footage from that night shows.

Three others arrived together shortly after him: a black woman, a white man in his forties and a black man with a limp. As the tape shows, at some point within minutes of sitting down, and before the others arrived, Rivera stops moving.

Unlike the security guard, who can be seen walking through the waiting area several times, the three "patients" immediately recognize that Rivera is in trouble. At first, they spread out around the room and sit in separate chairs. Then, slowly, one by one, they move closer to him, shifting from one chair to the next. Like the seats at my hospital, the ones in this waiting room are plastic and welded together in a bus-station-bench-like arrangement. They are a soothing aqua blue; some hospital designers have done their best to use relaxing color schemes to bring down the tension in these stress-filled areas.

Eventually, one of the men sidles up next to Rivera and sits. By now, the three of them are clustered around the not-moving man in one of the ER's U-shaped seating arrangements. The man sitting next to Rivera pauses, peering closely at his face, and then slowly slides the watch from his wrist. Rivera doesn't move. The man inspects the watch and then passes it on to his male compatriot. The woman looks on and then, furtively, peeks around.

Another man was in the ER waiting room that night. He saw the crime and, obviously outraged, summoned the guard. The robbers fled with the watch. Once the security response was activated, someone caught on to the fact that Rivera was in real medical trouble, and medics arrived quickly, but too late. The witness quotes a responding doctor as having taken one look at Rivera and said, "He's [expletive]ed." The three opportunists were eventually arrested. All turned out to be homeless, with prior records of drug- and alcohol-related arrests. It was subsequently determined that Rivera had suffered a heart attack, and a hospital spokesman acknowledged that the ER staff had not followed company policy requiring periodic checks on patients.

According the American Hospital Association, the total number of emergency room visits increased from 85 to 100 million between 1990 and 1999 in the United States, and many hospitals have been forced to expand their emergency departments. The very term *emergency room* is obviously hopelessly outdated. While hospitals may have had a single emergency *room* in the early part of the last century, by my father's era in the 1960s there was an emergency *ward*, with several curtained bays along each side of a corridor in the basement. In that era, an ambulance would roll in a couple of times a day with a sick patient.

For many hospitals today, this hospital entry point might best be described as an emergency *maw*—like the feeding aperture of a baleen whale—through which large volumes of patients are filtered more or less continuously. Many are treated and later expelled through that same orifice, while others are sucked into the entrails of the hospital, like krill, where they are digested in one fashion or another. Some leave cured. Others move on to long-term facilities in ambulances. And some, of course, eventually leave feet first.

While many patients typically have to wait hours before being seen in the emergency maw, the reason that they're there in the first place putting up with all of that inconvenience is often because it would take a much longer time to be seen by their own doctors. It's not unusual for friends of mine to tell me that their doctor is scheduled months in advance, and to ask if I could intervene to help move up the appointment for some unscheduled problem. We don't really have a good mechanism in modern health care to service the subacute issue. As a result, people go to the ER with colds, earaches, sore throats, belly pains, headaches and fever. Once upon a time, these problems would have been handled by a general practitioner.

The term *triage* originated from principles established during the Napoleonic wars by a French doctor named Dominique Jean Larrey, who was Napoleon's surgeon-in-chief. Extraordinarily innovative, he adapted the French "flying artillery" carts to double duty as "flying ambulances" in which trained crews "flew" across the battlefield gathering up wounded and dead. Darting through bullets, Larrey became so well known to his enemy— the English Duke of Wellington—that the duke ordered his troops not to fire in the direction of what he called that "brave man" with "the courage and devotion of an age that is no longer ours."[2]

Larrey also developed some of the first field hospitals and established the first rules for equitable triage, treating wounded soldiers according to the severity of their injuries rather than their social order, military rank or even their nationality. His services were highly valued by Napoleon himself, who promoted him to the rank of Baron and said, "If the army ever erects a monument to express its gratitude, it should do so in honor of Larrey."[3]

Baron Larrey was eventually captured by the Prussian army and condemned to death. Fortunately, he was recognized by a German surgical colleague who pled his case. Larrey treated both his own *and* enemy soldiers throughout his career; at one point he even saved the life of the son of a Prussian field marshal. Fortunate that someone recognized him and remembered the medical care he had provided to the Prussian soldier, he was eventually pardoned and released back to the French. Larrey died in his seventies after a long civilian medical career. His triage system was eventually formalized and refined during subsequent wars, and many triage variants have now been codified in different countries.

Patients who are expected to die regardless of treatment are variously termed "expectant" in the U.S. military system, "beyond urgency" by the French and "lost" in Finland. The triage function is typically performed by some type of medic. The French, for example, use the term *medecin trieur*, which translates to "sorter doctor," to refer to the physician in a forward army hospital who determines how best to allocate resources among the wounded.

Triage has evolved over the years, and while it is still practiced in military hospitals in today's seemingly endless wars, a civilian triage approach has developed in emergency rooms and urgent care clinics. The common denominator for each of these venues is the unexpected, unplanned nature of the patient visits. The *trieur* faces a continuous stream of patients with different conditions of varying severity and sorts them into "buckets": the urgent, the routine and the lost. The *trieur* must ask, "Does the guy with pain in his stomach have gas pains, an evolving heart attack or a nail in his stomach?" I've seen patients arrive with the same chief complaint of "stomach pain" who ended up having each of these problems. Above all else, the triage job requires experience and judgment. In fact, experienced *trieurs* believe that what they do is among the most intuitive of medical activities, one that absolutely requires human judgment. But perhaps they're wrong.

I recently saw this taped interaction between a *triaguer* (in this case an androgynous female), a mother and her sick young son.

"Hi. Thanks for coming," says the medical worker, greeting a mother with her 5-year-old son. "Are you here for the child or yourself?"

"The boy," the mother replies. "He has diarrhea."

"Oh no. Sorry to hear that," she says, looking down at the boy.

The nurse asks the mother about other symptoms, including fever ("slight") and abdominal pain ("he hasn't been complaining").

She turns again to the boy. "Has your tummy been hurting?"

"Yes," he answers.[4]

After a few more directed questions, the medical clinician indicates that she's not concerned at this point, and schedules a follow-up appointment a few days hence.

As the mother and child walk away, the boy peers curiously back over his shoulder at the computer screen from which the nurse spoke; she's not at all what he expected. "She" is actually a medical avatar designed at Microsoft Research, a computer and robotics laboratory on the Microsoft campus in Redmond, Washington.

This medical avatar was the product of a Microsoft demonstration project headed by Eric Horvitz, an artificial intelligence pioneer. The avatar has the ability to see, hear, speak, reason and learn, and had to perform a number of discrete tasks while it engaged in the interaction described above. First, it had to determine with which of the two humans to engage; note that "her" first question was addressed to the mother. Using clues like physical size, head orientation and scene analysis, the avatar had determined that the pair represented a parent and child, and it appropriately addressed the older, larger person.

The avatar then used a mix of acoustic and visual cues to determine what's being said and by whom. While analyzing the patient, the avatar was simultaneously keeping track of her own status. For example, when speaking, her indicators for "HasFloor," "IsListening," and "InConversation" are all set to be "True," because she was engaged in all of those actions concurrently. Similarly, based on eye contact and head position, she's set the "Goal" status indicator for the mother, whom she's labeled as "Actor 0," to "GetAssistance." She's also set the mother's "Activity" status to "Interacting" and the "Role" indicator to "Caregiver." The young boy, "Actor 1," is also flagged by the avatar as "GetAssistance" and "Interacting" but *his* "Role" is "DxFocus," which means that he is the diagnostic target, or patient.

The avatar's-eye view of the scene, which can be accessed on the Microsoft Research website, shows a distorted, wide-angle view of the mother and child.[5] A moving rectangle tracks and frames the heads of both as they look at the camera, each other and back. A red dot in the center of the frame indicates the center of each face, and a green arrow indicates the direction of their gaze. The red dot, rectangle and arrows dance constantly in front of and around the faces of the two humans, like the automated tracking systems of a fighter jet's heads-up display. Obviously a significant amount of background computing is going on continuously, to isolate the human head from the background image and track the eyes.

Although the avatar's speech is halting and distinctly non-human, a lot like the synthesized voice of the physicist Stephen Hawking, her head and facial expressions were modeled after a human female Microsoft employee. Andrea, an engaging receptionist at the computer company, was asked to model a series of facial expressions and head positions, such as those characterizing happiness, sorrow, surprise and amusement, to create a databank for the avatar to draw on when required.[6] During the course of her interaction with the mother and child, the computerized triage nurse uses several of these expressions.

The avatar uses another set of software to construct the dialogue with which she responds to the child's parent. Basically, she analyzes what she's heard and then uses a computer algorithm to construct the correct response, which is vocalized with a speech synthesizer. Here, too, there's some awkwardness in the sentence construction and word choice. She asks the child, for example, "Have you felt nawwsheuss?" After a pause, he answers, "I don't know," either because he just doesn't know the word nauseous, or perhaps because he can't understand her pronunciation of it.

Unfazed, she presses on, asking the mother, "Has your child been vomiting at all?" When the boy indicates that his stomach's been bothering him, the avatar parses that information and determines that an expression of sympathy is appropriate. She says, "Oh, I'm really sorry. I hope it—will—feel—bet-ter—soon." But she's not entirely stilted; in fact the avatar actually has an engaging little verbal tic, periodically throwing in a "Let's see" or "OK" while she mentally scrolls through a list of potential answers. She even blinks.

Based on the responses to her questions, the avatar uses a built-in probability system to determine what's most likely to be going on with the boy medically. Her underlying software relies on a logical construct first described by an eighteenth century clergyman and mathematician named Thomas Bayes. He realized that one way to predict the probability of something occurring in the future was to work with data about what happened in the past when the same situation occurred. So, for example, while it would be impossible to know with certainty what color ball I might pick out of a covered basket of red, green and blue balls, I could make pretty accurate predictions based on a sufficient number of prior trials.

If I *knew* there were twenty green balls and ten of each of the other colors in the basket, I'd know that there was a 50-percent chance that I'd pull out a green ball on any given pick. But even if I didn't know the composition for sure, or even how many balls were in the basket in the first place, it's pretty likely that after a thousand picks (i.e., prior trials), I'd know that I'd picked a green ball 50 percent of the time and a red or blue one 25 percent of the remaining times. I could then use those prior trial results to predict that there would be a 50-percent chance that any given ball I'd pick in the future would be green (assuming, of course, that the balls were randomly jumbled after each pick).

This same approach can be used to guide medical decision making. Based on knowledge about prior probabilities relating to diseases and tests, a human clinician (or a computer avatar) can make reasonably well-informed decisions about the likelihood that a new patient has a problem requiring immediate assessment or, alternatively, that there's nothing that can't wait for a scheduled visit. For example, a Bayesian logic system could help guide decision making relating to whether or not antibiotics should be prescribed for a urinary tract infection.

Anne Cervantes went to her primary care doctor, Dr. Terry Borges, after several days of burning on urination and a sense of urgency, typical symptoms of a bacterial urinary tract infection (UTI) in a young woman. An experienced clinician, Borges knew that these symptoms make it pretty likely that she had a treatable infection, but he wanted to be more certain. Fortunately there are some inexpensive and quick tests he can use to push his degree of certainty in one direction or another. The leukocyte esterase test, for example, tests the urine for an enzyme made by white blood cells, the inflammation fighters. A urine leukocyte esterase test can determine whether or not that enzyme is in the urine. If positive, it suggests that there is inflammatory activity somewhere in the urinary system, including the kidneys, bladder or urethra.

If Anne's test was positive for leukocyte esterase, it would increase Dr. Borges's suspicion that she had a UTI. A negative test, on the other hand, would decrease that likelihood and would have prompted him to seek out other causes for her symptoms. Similarly, the urine nitrite test, another urine assay, turns positive in the presence of a bacterial waste product, which increases the probability of her having a bacterial infection, while a negative test suggests a non-traditional bacterial source, like chlamydia.

A typical clinician like Dr. Borges doesn't actually think in terms of numerical probabilities, like the odds with the balls in a bucket, but the outcomes of tests like the esterase and nitrite-dip tests *can* be distilled down into real numbers that are digestible by a computer, allowing a computerized avatar to act like a primary care provider. The leukocyte esterase test, for example, has a sensitivity of 0.7, a specificity of 0.8 and likelihood ratios of 4.9 if positive and 0.3 if negative. The nitrite test, on the other hand, has a sensitivity of 0.5, specificity of 0.98, a positive likelihood ratio of almost 30.0 and negative ratio of 0.5. By now, I suspect you're wondering what these numbers mean.

The *sensitivity* of a test quantifies the fraction of those with a disease correctly identified by that test as having it. So both the esterase and the nitrite tests are reasonably good for the diagnosis of urinary infections, with sensitivities of around 75 percent. The *specificity,* on the other hand, is the fraction of those *without* the disease correctly identified by the test as *not* having it. A highly sensitive test, then, is very good at picking up patients with the disease, but it may also have false positives; in other words, it's good for screening. A very specific test, on the other hand, is almost certain to be right if it's positive but may miss some true positives. The nitrite test is very specific, getting it right almost 100 percent of the time if it's positive. The *likelihood ratio* for a positive test, which incorporates both the sensitivity and the specificity, indicates how much more likely you are to have the disease with a positive result than someone with a negative result. The same is true in reverse for a negative likelihood ratio. So a patient with a positive nitrite test is about 30 times more likely to have a bacterial urinary infection than someone with a negative test.

The actual numbers don't really matter so much. Nor do the terms. What's more important is the fact that, given enough numbers of this kind—enough information about patients and tests and confirmed diseases—a computer can be programmed to navigate its way to a place very similar to where a doctor would, based on the same information. In reality, the data an experienced doctor works with are past encounters, and a computer can be programmed to use data from past encounters in the form of experimental outcomes from research. The doctor arrives at his diagnosis based on his own individual intuition; a computer arrives at the same diagnosis based on the aggregated experience of many patient encounters distilled into numbers representing sensitivity, specificity and likelihood ratios. But with more and more accurate information about large numbers of patients, the computer can eventually begin to behave more and more like an experienced doctor.

When Anne came to Dr. Borges's office, she described her symptoms. He asked her to provide a urine sample, which the nurse tested using a dipstick. The urine dipstick is a strip of plastic with a number of pale-pastel indicator dyes arrayed along one end, which is submerged in the sample. The indicators test for the urine's acidity and the presence or level of glucose, protein, blood, leukocyte esterase and nitrites. The acid test is essentially pH dye, like the paper used in high school laboratories; the dye indicator turns somewhere between orange and blue based on how acid or alkaline the urine is. The glucose indicator, on the other hand, changes from a yellow color through progressively darker blues to brown in the presence of the higher glucose levels that one might find in diabetic or some pregnant patients. The blood indicator turns from a yellow to progressively bluer shades, depending on the amount of blood or hemoglobin in the sample. Abnormal amounts of protein in the urine, which are often found in a patient with kidney disease, change the protein indicator from a yellow to a greenish blue. The leukocyte esterase test turns purple on exposure to enzymes released by active white blood cells. And the nitrite test turns from white to pink if there are bacterial by-products in the urine.

When Anne's urine was tested with the dipstick, the blood, protein, esterase and nitrite tests all came up positive: blue, green-blue, purple and pink—which was exactly what one expects in a bacterial urinary tract infection where there is a lot of inflammation. Dr. Borges prescribed an antibiotic for Anne and also sent the urine off for a bacterial culture as a precaution. Unfortunately, many bacteria today are increasingly resistant to standard antibiotics; if Anne didn't respond to the first drug, Borges would know which stronger antibiotic to use next based on the outcome of the culture, which would take a couple of days to grow. Of course the advantage to prescribing something immediately is that if the first-line drug works, Anne will feel better sooner.

Anne's problem and her medical interaction with Dr. Borges represent a routine encounter for a common medical problem. The patient's complaints and the doctor's response are very straightforward and could one day be handled by a descendant of the Microsoft medical avatar, perhaps even one located in a kiosk at a pharmacy or company medical clinic. With something this simple, there's really no need for a doctor or even a human to be involved; the computer could prescribe the antibiotic. This is admittedly a radical proposal, but certainly no more radical than the idea of turning an airplane full of people over to an autopilot.

While the idea of having a conversation about your medical problems with an avatar on a screen seems alien to many of us today, automated speech analysis is creeping into our lives at an increasing pace. We've all interacted with a telephone company's automated operators, and companies like Google, Microsoft and Nokia have added "search-by-voice capabilities" to their products. Computer scientists expect substantial progress over the coming years in speech recognition and synthesis. And they're also progressing with artificially intelligent systems.

The same research team at Microsoft that developed the avatar has developed a product called SmartPhlow designed to identify potential traffic surprises. The system is a traffic-forecasting service that uses the vast amounts of "experimental" data that are increasingly available to us to predict when something surprising is about to happen with traffic flow in a congested city like Seattle.

SmartPhlow wasn't designed so much to identify traffic jams. It was designed to predict *surprising* traffic situations, such as better-than-usual traffic flow in a typically congested location or an unexpected jam where traffic usually flows smoothly. While traffic flow would seem to have little to do with medical care, the same sorts of tools can be applied to both to permit modeling. The Microsoft team started with years of data about traffic flow by time-of-day and correlated it with all sorts of things that typically impact it, like accidents, weather, holidays and sporting events.

By dividing each day's data into 15-minute chunks, and by road segments, they developed a very detailed picture of baseline traffic. The team then went back to identify traffic events, good or bad, that deviated significantly from the baseline—the surprises—and focused on them. These surprises, they assumed, would be of interest to the experienced Seattle driver who already knows about the *usual* choke points around the city.

Because they had a lot of very detailed data, the SmartPhlow team was able to look back to the period 30 minutes *before* a surprise event occurred to identify any subtle premonitory patterns that might be used to predict *future* surprises. They then used Bayesian algorithms, based directly on Thomas Bayes's work back in the mid-1700s, to calculate the probability, based on prior experience, that a surprise would happen in the future.

Another group from Microsoft Research approached the city traffic problem with an entirely different method. Recognizing the shortcomings of traditional global-positioning-system (GPS)-based navigation systems, the researchers who designed this project, called T-Drive, hypothesized that they could find a faster way to navigate the streets of China's choked cities. They attached GPS sensors to over 30,000 cabs and tracked them as the cabbies went about their business. With the help of sophisticated mathematical algorithms, they were able to capitalize on the resulting combination of human and machine intelligence to determine which routes were consistently chosen and which were avoided. After a three-month period of data gathering, they created a model in which drivers were consistently able to save about 5 minutes on what would ordinarily have been a half hour-drive. And while it might not be intuitively obvious at first, this same kind of analysis can be done in medicine to design "best practices."

As we get better at accurately labeling diseases, and tracking the progress of the disease with lots of data from a variety of sensors, we'll eventually have all of the tools to reproduce the T-Drive project. By labeling a given patient with the diagnosis of community-acquired pneumonia, we will know both the origin and destination of the disease. The origin, of course, is the patient's situation at the time of diagnosis, and the destination is "healthy." Once we've acquired lots of data about lots of patients and their treatment regimens, which are like the routes selected by skilled cabbies, we'll know which ones work best. The winning regimens will be designated *best practices*. And, as with route-finding programs, there may be a variety of alternative best practices depending on whether one scores by least cost, shortest time to wellness or other variables.

Imagine a patient in an intensive care unit or operating room who was admitted with a medical problem that's pretty well understood and has a predictable course, like that of a routine coronary artery bypass patient. Then assume that we develop a lot of information for lots of similar patients who've had bypass surgery about things like heart rate, blood pressure, respiratory rate and lab values, and that we segment this data into discrete time periods, like a nurse does when he records vital signs. With enough information, we could eventually develop a very accurate picture of what expected behavior looks like and then compare the course of any new patient to that template. This would allow us to identify outliers—"surprise" patients—who deviate from the norm and develop unexpected trouble. Using the T-Drive approach, we'll know what treatments work best. Then we can look back, just like the SmartPhlow team did to determine what was going on in the minutes or hours ahead of an unexpected turn for the worse to identify premonitory patterns allowing us to *predict* when a patient is about to get into trouble. In fact, some work has already been done along these lines.

In 2009, a group of researchers from Virginia Commonwealth University School of Medicine published a paper describing their use of "multivariate Bayesian models trained with machine learning in conjunction with rule-based time-series statistical techniques" to predict patient status in the intensive care unit.[7] In other words, they set out to create an intelligent monitoring system to predict when ICU patients are improving or declining. They used data, including the patient age, gender, diagnosis, blood pressure, temperature, heart rate and arterial oxygen saturation. It turned out that the behavior of a single patient versus their own baseline was a better predictor of future behavior than behavior versus the average.

The Microsoft emergency room avatar was designed as a proof-of-concept experiment. There are several independent but converging technology trends suggesting that we may see smart, robotic health-care providers in our hospitals and homes in the foreseeable future. The first trend is the dramatic increase in the amount of real electronic data we're accumulating about real patients. We used to have to rely on narrative case reports and limited data sets to describe specific diseases, but with the advent of continuous physiologic monitors, genomics and proteomics (the study of how proteins and enzymes affect health) we will soon be able to make very exact descriptions of diseases. And we'll be able to program those descriptions into computers. A second critical and related trend is the dramatic advances in our ability to use computer vision, hearing, speech and other senses to reproduce human interactions. The final element is robotics.

I recently attended a mobile-health summit featuring an interview with Bill Gates, whose recent interests and efforts have turned to improving the health of patients in impoverished countries. An interviewer asked him what he thought would be the most important technological contributor to medical care in the near future. His answer surprised me. He said that, based on what was happening in laboratories around the world, robotics would be the key driver in the care of certain populations such as the elderly, the pregnant and the injured. He went on to hedge that answer a bit, admitting that we'll see dramatic advances in drug design as well, as we come to understand the three-dimensional structure of critical proteins, but reiterated his projection about robotics.

The convergent opportunities inherent in massive data sets, human–computer interaction techniques and robotics will result in the development of smart, experienced, interactive robotic assistants that can facilitate all sorts of things humans don't like to do or do poorly. One of the first places they'll be deployed is in the provision of medical care.

PART IV

NEW MODELS OF CARE

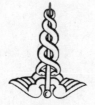

In the final section of the book, I'll introduce you to a loser in medicine's dog-eat-dog trenches. We'll see the medical food chain, up close, and the frantic competition for rations and water that will inevitably occur as once-lush monetary watering holes dry up. We'll watch as medical care evolves, as new techniques emerge and medical specialties that once played a subservient support role become fitter and cannibalize more complacent siblings. Cardiologists don scrubs and steal the bacon of their surgical counterparts. Nurses don long white coats and a doctoral degree, directly challenging what were once the domains of physicians.

And entrepreneurs have created novel models of medical care that threaten to disrupt existing paradigms, just as digital photography disrupted and displaced acetate film and cars displaced their equine predecessors. The patient seems to have gotten lost in the stampede of medical innovation over the past decades, as what was once a cradle-to-grave relationship between a patient and her doctor has fragmented into a series of episodic managements of medical crises. But the patient-centered medical home is a model offering the promise of a return to a more coherent and constant relationship between a patient and his team of providers, while acknowledging the need for technologies that improve care without dehumanizing it.

CHAPTER 14

SURVIVAL OF
THE FIT

Each cadaver in my medical school anatomy class had four students assigned to it. The assignments were by alphabetical order, so there was no question of buddies grouping up to share the admittedly ghoulish work. The guys at my table, and it was all men only through happenstance, had last names starting with Ha and He. Everyone had his own dissection kit consisting of an assortment of scissors, tweezers, hemostats (stainless steel surgical clamps), probes and scalpels, each with its separate slot in a canvas roll-up bag. There were also boxes of gloves all around, and we all wore blue plastic smocks. Everyone inevitably ended up smelling like formaldehyde by the end of the day, regardless of the degree to which she participated in the dissection, and there was a whole range of participation. Some loved dissection, some didn't care much one way or the other, and some really hated it.

We had all arrived at medical school in a relatively undifferentiated state; we were all just generic premedical students. But the Gross Anatomy lab started immediately, and the students rapidly began to differentiate into one medical type or another; some liked to work with their hands, others with their minds.

Anatomy was a great culling mechanism, in that it tended to split the "doers" from the "thinkers." Every day, as I looked down the aisle of cadavers surrounded by students, the same people tended to be doing the dissection while their less action-minded partners looked on. At our table, for example, one of the He's and one of the Ha's were dissectors, while the other two preferred to leaf through a well-thumbed, formaldehyde-covered copy of *Grey's Anatomy* and point out anatomical landmarks. A wizened old gray-beard doctor, like the retired Scottish general surgeon who taught the class, could probably have stood back and looked around, mentally dividing the room into surgeons and non-surgeons, and he would have been pretty accurate. Within a year, many of us were beginning to figure out which medical kingdom we belonged to; the cognitively oriented students knew they were different from their procedurally oriented brethren.

My good friend Paul was the He at my anatomy table who liked to use a scalpel. He liked using *any* kind of instrument or tool, and he was very good with them. Unlike the rest of us, forceps and a scalpel already looked comfortable in his hands on the first day of class. Like me, Paul was the son of a doctor; his father was a urologist who practiced into his nineties. Paul and I both had backed our way into medicine after exploring alternatives, giving us a common bond as we were both a couple of years older than the majority of the class.

We both had majored in fine arts rather than premedical disciplines in college. College pictures show Paul as a bearded baby boomer who happened to be an extremely skilled woodworker. He caught his wife, Mary Lou, a talented graphic designer, very much off guard when he decided on a radical career change after they were married for a few years. He announced that he had decided to go to medical school.

Paul had started his post-graduate career making beautiful pieces of furniture with tools like the plane, lathe and wood chisel. Once he entered medical school, it wasn't a huge leap to the use of equally sharp and precise surgical instruments. It was immediately apparent to the rest of us, as well as to our Scottish instructor, that he'd eventually enter one of the surgical disciplines. When he later decided to go into orthopedics, none of us were surprised. In fact, "orthopods" use many of the same tools that carpenters do, including hammers, chisels, drills and screws. Paul was fortunate in that he didn't have to struggle too much with his career choice. Others, like me, did.

For a medical student, the choices among specialties can be daunting. There are a huge number of variables in choosing a medical career pathway, and each specialty has a range of sub-specialty options to go with it. The medical student typically has far too little data to make a well-informed choice when the time comes.

Like most professional schools, medical school offers a mix of core curricula and electives. Core areas of study include microbiology, histology (the study of body tissues), normal and abnormal physiology, immunology and genetics. These areas are usually completed during the first two years of the four-year curriculum. The third year is devoted to what are called *clinical clerkships* (during which the medical student first has significant patient care responsibilities) in the base disciplines that a medical student must become familiar with to become an effective physician in any specialty. Internal medicine, surgery, pediatrics, family medicine, obstetrics and gynecology, anesthesiology, neurology and emergency medicine are all basic rotations, as are ophthalmology, orthopedics and ear, nose and throat. Non-clinical areas like radiology and pathology are woven through these core patient-care rotations. The fourth year is set aside for electives in which a student can focus on areas that may complement or inform her choice of residencies, although by then there's very little time left to explore.

So it is only at the conclusion of the third year of medical school that a student has gotten enough exposure to the broad range of medical specialties to realistically even begin to decide whether he be fish or fowl, as it were. By the fourth year, the typical medical student has had no more than a month's time in each of the specialties, and his experience is typically skewed in one way or another. For example, the core internal medicine rotation at many medical schools is designed to expose the student to *hospitalized* patients with the kinds of diseases that a *hospital*-based internist, such as the hospitalist I described in an earlier chapter, might deal with—like pneumonia, out-of-control diabetes or chest pain. The problem is that most internists actually do most of their work in a medical office, *not* a hospital, so the medical student may have an inaccurate picture of internal medicine as a career.

As the son of an internist and someone who essentially grew up in a doctor's office, I should have understood this. But I made the same error that a lot of medical students do and started down one career path only to realize a couple of years later that I had made a mistake and needed to make an emergency mid-course correction. I started in an internal medicine residency because I liked the detective work involved in diagnosing diseases. And I actually loved what I did until one memorable day when I was seeing a patient in an outpatient clinic at the Palo Alto veterans' hospital.

My patient had arrived with his wife, and the two of them were sitting across from me in chairs, side by side, as I sat at one of those big governmental-green metal desks writing notes in the chart. I went through my usual questions.

"What brought you here?"

"How long have you had that?"

"Any family history of…?"

Everything went pretty smoothly, at first, although I noticed that the wife jumped in with a lot of the answers before her somewhat passive husband got a chance to open his mouth.

Then I asked whether he had hemorrhoids—a standard, but awkward part of the Review of Systems—and the answer changed my life. The missus was able to answer this one, too, without even a pause.

She allowed as how he *did* indeed have hemorrhoids, that they were big, and that they sometimes protruded—"hung out" as she put it—after he had a bowel movement. She said he sometimes actually had to "push them back in" sometimes just to be comfortable. He nodded along passively as she answered for him.

I can still see that couple in my mental scrapbook, and it was at exactly that moment that I realized I wanted to do something other than office-based medicine for the rest of my life—despite the fact that I'd already invested a year and a half in training to be an internist. I didn't ever want to be in the position of trying to work through another conversation like that again. Fairly or unfairly, those 15 minutes came to symbolize what I feared would become many years of similar encounters. I say this with the greatest respect for my colleagues who do this every day, including my own internist—it just wasn't me. I did finish my residency in internal medicine, my father's profession, but eventually went on to become an anesthesiologist and critical care doctor. And I've never again had to deal that directly, or indirectly as in this case, with hemorrhoids.

There are many ways to approach the decision about which medical specialty to enter, and the decision is so important that books have been written about it. The University of Virginia's medical school actually has an online test designed to tell students which career choice might be best for them. The UVA online test assesses the answers to a series of 130 questions, asking the respondent whether, for example, they tend to be a doer rather than a thinker or comfortable with long-term rather than immediate results.

The underlying engine for these questions is the Myers-Briggs Type Indicator (or MBTI), which is a psychometric questionnaire originally designed to help women entering the workforce during World War II to determine what fields would best suit them. Since the mid-1900s, the MBTI instrument has been adapted for more general-purpose use as a screening tool to help individuals determine where they fall in the proprietary Myers-Briggs four-dimensional personality matrix.

The first axis is *extraversion* versus *introversion*. The MBTI attempts to determine whether an individual prefers to focus on the outer action-oriented world or the world within, where concepts and ideas live. The *sensing* versus *intuition* axis evaluates the way in which someone processes data: do they focus on basic objective information or add a layer of interpretation and meaning? A tendency to act logically and impersonally in decision making, like the *Star Trek* character Spock, scores highly on the *thinking* end of the scale, while someone who prefers to look at the people involved and the impact of special circumstances is more of a *feeler*. Finally, individuals who are more comfortable in an orderly, structured environment, where they can control events around them, are *judgers,* while those with a tendency towards a flexible and spontaneous, adaptive way of life show a bias towards *perceiving.*

Using these axes, an MBTI expert (and as one might predict, there is a certification in this field) might describe someone with Extrovert-Sensing-Thinking-Judging biases—an ESTJ type—as having a predilection for leadership and managing others. For example, air-traffic controllers are likely to have ESTJ personalities. On the other hand, an ESTJ's opposite, the INFP, tends to avoid the spotlight and maintain a reserved posture—rarely, if ever, finding her way into a CEO role.

While these classifications aren't absolute predictors of one's future, according to the Myers and Briggs Foundation, "Whatever the circumstances of your life, the understanding of type can make your perceptions clearer, your judgments sounder and your life closer to your heart's desire."[1] Isabel Briggs Myers wrote these words and, with her mother Katherine Cook Briggs, developed the personality inventory based on Carl Jung's psychological work.

Carl Jung published the book *Psychological Types* in 1921. And Briggs and Myers became American "type watchers" almost immediately after the book was translated into English in 1923, eventually developing a pen-and-pencil version of the questionnaire that has now been translated into many languages and applied to a variety of general and specific applications, including the one offered by the University of Virginia to confused medical students looking for a specialty.

The University of Virginia tool has its basis in a study originally performed by Isabel Briggs Myers at the George Washington University School of Medicine. She tested approximately 5,000 medical students to determine their MBTI personality type and how type influenced career preferences. This work was eventually published as a monograph in 1977 and showed how medical students rated the attractiveness of different fields while they were still in medical school, based on an abbreviated version of their personality type. The findings were interesting.[2]

Sensor/Thinkers found child psychiatry extremely unappealing, while their opposites, Intuitive/Feelers loved the field. The Intuitive/Feelers on the other hand, hated anesthesiology, my field, and orthopedics. To be fair, these tests were done on medical students 40 years ago and are now probably hopelessly out of date as all of these fields have changed substantially over that interval. The study only tells us about what first-year medical students thought of specialties they hadn't yet experienced—their uninformed impressions. As an example, the Intuitive/Feeler med students who liked Child Psychiatry also liked Neurosurgery, whereas in my experience, neurosurgeons couldn't possibly be more different from adolescent psychiatrists.

A more recent study used the MBTI instrument to analyze medical students' predilections for choosing between (1) primary and non-primary care residencies, (2) family medicine as opposed to internal medicine or pediatrics and (3) surgical versus non-surgical, non-primary care specialties. The authors found that Extroverted/Thinker types, what Myers and Briggs would categorize as the "overseers" and "chiefs," ended up selecting action-oriented disciplines like surgery, while Introverted/Feelers, the "artists" and "dreamers," tended to go into primary care specialties like family medicine, internal medicine and pediatrics.

As the authors of this more recent study put it: "This finding is not surprising in that primary care is highly service-oriented; money and prestige are not as likely to be motivating factors for primary practitioners. The rewards of long-term relationships with patients and families are consistent with preferences for feeling and introversion."[3] The study's findings don't seem that surprising. Medicine is attractive to lots of different types of people because it's a very diverse field. There's room for the nurturing pediatrician, the demanding surgeon, the watchful anesthesiologist and the inquisitive pathologist.

Species in an ecosystem either find hospitable niches or become food for other species and die off; and medical students usually sort themselves out pretty effectively into fields that suit their personalities, as per some medical "Natural Order." As any parent knows, children first learn to sort themselves out instinctively on the playground. This development of pecking orders is not something that's susceptible to legislation; you can't tell an alpha male or female *not* to be one, any more than you can tell an omega kid to be an alpha. Playground supervisors know this. But the people who conceived of the medical reform efforts in the 1990s didn't. These guys thought it would be a good idea to put nice guys in charge of the gladiators and deployed the Gatekeeper Model of managed care.

The gatekeeper concept puts the primary care doctor, typically a general or family practitioner, pediatrician or internist, in the role of bouncer. In order to be seen by a specialist, the primary care provider had to approve a referral. Insurance companies in the 1990s liked this concept as a method of cost containment for a bunch of reasons. It took the burden of refusal off the company and put it in the hands of a doctor. What, they asked, could be wrong with placing the responsibility for coordination of care, access to care and continuity in the hands of the very people who espoused those principles—the primary care doctors?

The hidden beauty of this arrangement, of course, is that by placing a few individuals in charge, insurers developed a point at which they could place an economic lever. They could, they thought, manage costs by managing the gatekeepers. Gatekeepers who were too liberal in referrals to specialists were penalized in some way, while the "better" gatekeepers—the ones who kept costs down—were rewarded. A few initial experiments with the model looked promising, but the problems with gatekeeping in real practice quickly became evident after this approach became widely adopted. As one publication put it:

> Control of the "referral gate" to specialty care often is a lose-lose proposition for primary care providers in managed care arrangements. If primary care physicians approve referrals to specialists too

freely, they risk a reduction in their capitation rate or depletion of the fund reserved for specialty care and procedures. Also specialists may complain about referrals for conditions that they think the primary care provider should have managed alone. Conversely, when primary care physicians infrequently open the gate to specialty care, patients may believe their physicians are denying them necessary care. Some plans reduce the primary care physician's capitation rate when patients are dissatisfied. These opposing forces squeeze the primary care physician who is trying to meet patient needs at a reasonable cost.[4]

There was yet another critical force that came into play with gatekeeping, which was the specialist's ability to take potshots at primary care doctors when they missed a diagnosis or mismanaged a patient. Specialty journals of the later 1990s are full of studies showing that the specialists who subscribed to their professional journal handled their patients' problems better than primary doctors did. This isn't too surprising, of course. Most of the readers of *American Rifleman* probably believe that they can do a better job of handling inner-city violence than gun-control advocates can.

Of course, the real problem with putting primary care doctors in charge of the playground is that, by so doing, we're inverting the "Natural Medical World Order" by putting Intuitive/Feelers in charge of Extroverted/Thinkers, which is a profoundly unnatural arrangement. Many medical staffs consist in some part of extremely talented but socially stunted individuals who were busily studying in medical school during the years that their non-medical contemporaries were out in the world, developing adult social skills. Playground supervisors and prison guards would feel right at home in any doctor's lunchroom, immediately recognizing the assembled personality types and their likely specialties.

The fact of the matter is that humans, like almost every other animal, innately *get* who should be in charge of whom, and they don't *like it* when the wrong guy is arbitrarily put in charge. My youngest son, Callaghan, for example, goes ballistic, yelling, "You're not in charge of me!" when one of his twin brothers, Addison or Watson, oversteps some invisible but mutually understood authoritative boundary. The Western medical system has evolved to reward those assertive specialists who put in extra years of training to become authoritative experts in narrower fields than their touchy-feely primary-care brethren. While the latter are content with "the rewards of long-term relationships with patients and families," many of the former have found their way into procedurally oriented fields like surgery, interventional cardiology and ophthalmology.

The procedure doctors are the *doers*. They *like* to be in charge and in control. They *thrive* on immediate gratification, and they don't typically have the patience to put up with long-term patient-care relationships. For better or worse, Western medicine is currently structured to reward the ESTJ doers—the "proceduralists"—disproportionately over Intuitive/Feeler listeners. This asymmetry in rewards and personality types is what makes what will come next in health care so interesting. What will the doctors of the future do as medical resources become constrained? Who will survive and who won't?

The History Channel recently debuted a television series entitled *Life After People*. This apocalyptic show pictures the deteriorating skyscrapers, shaky bridges, vine-covered ball fields and the fate of various animal species that the show's producers believe will be left behind after mankind vacates the Earth—willingly or otherwise. Suffice it to say that, in their view, lapdogs, house cats and domesticated farm animals will disappear rather quickly, bite by bite, while the big, feral dogs will do just fine. These big dogs are the Extroverted/Thinkers of the animal kingdom. And while the future of medicine certainly won't be an apocalyptic life without patients, there *will* be a scramble, similar to the one envisioned in *Life After People*, in which the evolutionary fitness of various medical pursuits will be tested.

I recently interviewed a cardiac surgeon who wanted a job working entire weekends, day and night, Friday night through Monday morning, in one of our intensive care units. His story was an interesting cautionary tale about what evolutionarily unfit doctors can look forward to in the world of *Life after Health Care Reform*. Dr. Bryan Scherr (not his real name) had a blue-ribbon CV. He'd graduated from Yale University with a degree in physics and headed to Stanford University for medical school. Bryan had gone on to UCLA for an internship and back to Stanford for his surgical residency, eventually completing training in vascular and cardiothoracic surgery at UCLA and Stanford. Scherr had been schooled and trained at top American educational and medical institutions and went on to become a cardiac surgeon—one of the apex "predators" of the medical system. This guy was a poster-child ESTJ alpha male.

Dr. Scherr went on to enter a lucrative private practice in cardiac surgery in California, which he described to me saying: "It used to be that you could see patients on a Monday, bang out three or four hearts [by which he meant operations on patients needing coronary artery bypass grafting] a week and make a very good living, with time off to play golf." However, for reasons he didn't explain, his private practice broke up toward the end of 2008, so he tried some *locum tenens* work, wherein an itinerant surgeon substitutes for someone who is disabled or away. The Latin term *locum tenens* translates to "hold the place," and this is a common way of describing work done by wandering physicians like the one Scherr had become.

But placeholding is not a durable fiscal model, as he was soon to find out. Scherr tried to find a new cardiac surgical practice after his practice broke up, but those jobs are scarce today, even for new trainees. For the now 62-year-old Scherr, it was impossible to find cardiac surgical work, so he adapted and began to work taking care of patients other surgeons had operated on. He found part-time jobs in an intensive care unit in New York, and another in California, and he had applied to work at our unit in Philadelphia as well. At one point during the interview I asked him if he was planning on coming down from New York to Philadelphia, which is a manageable 90-minute train ride or slightly longer in a car. His answer stunned me. Scherr intended to commute from Los Angeles, 3,000 miles and a several-hour-longer ride away—albeit a commute that turned out, he said, to be not much more expensive than the train if he bought his tickets from an online discount ticket purveyor.

There in my office that day I had a 62-year-old, highly trained heart surgeon with no obvious disabilities who had at one point worked his way to the very top of a heap consisting entirely of people who'd been plucked from the tops of other heaps, only to be reduced to flying around the country working nighttime shifts in a series of ICUs between airplane rides. Scherr had come all the way from California to look at a job in which there was a very good possibility that he'd be up covering one crisis after another, more or less continuously for 60 hours at the ripe old age of 62. And we got *several* similar applications just like Scherr's for that job.

How, I asked myself, could this possibly have happened? It reminded me of those nature films where some once-proud king beast, perhaps missing just a few teeth or an antler, is up and ousted from the pack by a young, bold new competitor. If he survives the joust, he's then forced to wander the land, feeding off scraps and carcasses.

So, how *did* this happen? Well, it's conceivable there was some "issue" in Scherr's past that might not have been evident from his CV and prevented him from obtaining another surgical job, but I had no reason to believe this, and there are plenty of alternative explanations. Cardiac surgery was a once highly sought-after, lucrative field that seemed well worth the cost of years of training.

The average practicing cardiac surgeon has completed four years of college, four years of medical school and eight-and-a-half years of residency plus fellowship. He doesn't become a finished product until he's in his mid-thirties. Worse yet, according to a study of newly minted cardiac surgeons published recently, a significant proportion couldn't find a job when they finished.[5] The respondents started their *real* life with an average of $50,000 in debt. More than half would have counseled potential trainees to go into another field. And, perhaps most tellingly, nearly one quarter reported that they would not have chosen a career in cardiac surgery had they known when they started what the future would look like when they were done training. The landscape had changed dramatically in the interval.

The operations Bryan Scherr performed three or four times a week in his prime were probably a mix of heart valve replacements and coronary arterial bypass procedures, more popularly known as CABG or, in the layman's vernacular, cabbages. The first CABGs were done in the early 1960s by pioneers like Dr. Rene Favalaro, an Argentinian from humble beginnings who trained and began his medical career in South America but eventually emigrated to the United States and Ohio's famed Cleveland Clinic.

While a trainee, Favalaro became fascinated with the coronary circulation, which provides blood flow to the heart muscle. As is so often the case, "chance favor[ed] the prepared mind."[6] The Cleveland Clinic also had a large collection of x-rays showing the heart vessels of many patients. These angiograms had been performed by another cardiac pioneer, Dr. Mason Sones, the father of coronary angiography. Many of these angiograms showed blockages in heart vessels, and, in a brilliant insight, it occurred to Favalaro that one could divert, or bypass, blood flow around these blockages, using a vein harvested from the leg—the saphenous vein.

Favalaro became extremely successful and eventually established a medical foundation back in Argentina modeled after the Cleveland Clinic.

The Favalaro Foundation did extremely well for the quarter-century between 1975 and the year 2000, but then Argentina fell into a financial crisis. His foundation fell on hard times, and, despite Favalaro's petitions, the Argentine government refused to intervene to help. It folded. Devastated, Favalaro committed suicide by shooting himself in the heart, the very organ he'd done so much to heal during his life.

Bypass grafting has lived on, however, and it eventually revolutionized cardiac surgery. The operation eventually became so common that more than a million CABG operations were performed in the United States between 1988 and 2003. But, almost imperceptibly at first, something happened to change what had been a steadily increasing trend over the last few years of that 15-year period.

Most studies show that the number of CABGs peaked in about 1996. By this time, many ambitious community hospitals saw that the ability to advertise cardiac surgery as a service line represented an evolutionary edge over competitors. Whole teams were recruited to hospitals all over the United States during the early 1990s, including cardiologists, cardiac surgeons, the perfusionists who run heart-lung bypass machines and intensive care staffs. But an interesting thing happened over the three- or four-year span between 1996 and 1999. The overall number of CABGs started to decrease, subtly at first, but quite clearly by 1999—yet the number of new cardiac programs kept on increasing.

The community hospital administrators who were building these new programs hadn't cottoned to the fact that their food source was about to be in peril. By 1999, the majority of CABGs, by percentage, were being done at so-called *low-volume* hospitals, which typically have less-good outcomes. And because there were more programs doing CABGs every year while the number of patients needing them didn't increase at the same rate, each program was doing fewer of these surgeries than they had a few years earlier. The more experienced, *high-volume* programs were getting hit harder as patients were being siphoned off to new low-volume hospitals, and reimbursement rates were being cut by insurers. In effect, what had been boom times with a reliable food source for cardiac surgeons, and the dependent consultative medical and nursing specialties, all of a sudden went bust. This all happened about midway through the career of the now-itinerant Dr. Bryan Scherr.

So why did the number of CABG surgeries start to decline? Was it because we stopped eating Cheese-Whiz–covered fries that had been cooked in tasty trans fats? Were new cholesterol drugs working miraculous cures? Had everyone stopped smoking? In a word, no.

What really happened was that cardiologists got wise. For years they had been *diagnosing* patients with coronary disease, doing the angiograms, and then sending them off, one by one, to a prima donna cardiac *surgeon* who would "bang out" a few CABGs between golf games before retiring in his brand-new Mercedes to his multimillion-dollar home. The *cardiologist*, in turn, drove home hours later in his Honda to a much more modest, split-level home. During the commute, he perseverated about ways to level the playing field.

Then along came the revolutionary balloon coronary angioplasty, coronary roto-rooters, coronary vascular stents and increasingly sophisticated ways for a cardiologist to "operate" on the heart without ever picking up a scalpel. These innovative cardiologists developed clever new techniques allowing them to reopen blocked heart vessels *non-invasively*, thereby eliminating the need for cardiac surgery in all but the most complicated cases.

By the late 1990s, with these new techniques, cardiologists had in effect figured out a way to steal the cardiac surgeon's bacon. What ensued in many small hospitals over the succeeding decade was analogous to those televised scenes from the African veldt where some proud lion king is hunched down anxiously over the carcass of an animal that his queens have brought down and is surrounded by a pack of hungry, disrespectful hyenas. The dogs move ever closer, eyes sparkling in the night, making that eerie laughing sound that hyenas make. And in every show I've ever seen, the lion eventually gives it up as a bad job and skulks away.

Maybe, I said to myself as I ended my interview, *this* is what had happened to Dr. Bryan Scherr, the wandering cardiac surgeon. Maybe the routine CABGs that had kept him busy and wealthy in his 1990s-era private practice had just dried up as his one-time supporting-cast cardiologists began to handle more and more of them non-operatively.

When the designated hour was up, I thanked him for his time and moved on mentally to my next task. But he kept sitting there, on my couch, reminiscing wistfully about his residency at Stanford. Eventually I tried a power "interview-ender" move. I actually stood and reached out my hand to shake his. It didn't faze him a bit. He went right on talking. Scherr was back in his glory days and would do anything to avoid looking at the stark realities of a modern medicine that had passed him by. In this new era, for some professionals, it's already a dog-eat-dog world.

Gastroenterologists have figured out non-operative ways to remove gall-stones, cauterize bleeding ulcers and reshape the stomach to treat obesity—traditionally all things that a general surgeon would do during an operation under anesthesia. Cardiologists are now working on ways to repair and replace heart valves using catheters inserted through the blood vessels very much like the ones they use to put stents in the coronaries. They are thereby finding another way to do the work of, and bedevil, cardiac surgeons who have always done these operations while a patient is on cardiopulmonary bypass and then only after cutting open his chest. Radiologists, gastroenter-ologists and general surgeons all compete to do another procedure: placing a feeding tube through the skin into a patient's stomach. And a variety of different surgical specialists insert tracheostomy breathing tubes into the neck. Everybody wants to "own" their own procedure.

The ESTJ "doers" may see patients in the office in order to determine whether or not there is something to "do," but they really live for those moments when they are actually doing something with their hands. These are the physician kingdom's carnivore equivalents. They don't mind spilling blood or sawing bone. They like immediate gratification. They like to look at problems logically and impersonally and don't spend a lot of time on intu-ition. They like objectivity. They are extroverts and are not uncomfortable with being perceived as near godlike by their patients.

The opposites of the "doers" are the more meditative cognitive special-ists—the INFP "thinkers." Like my father, they actually enjoy listening to a patient's story and leafing through their mental library of previous cases to find a diagnosis that fits this case. The best way to compliment a thinker is to acknowledge a "good pick-up," praising his identification of some obscure but absolutely critical piece of information in a patient's database. Thinkers prefer not to be bloodied or soiled by contact with a patient, and they cringe at the sound of a bone saw. They don't mind watching the evolution of a problem over weeks, months or years. They pride their sense of intuition and recognize that the facts don't always tell the whole truth. They are com-fortable with uncertainty. The INFPs are introverts in the sense that they like the world of ideas and concepts, the inner world. And they have the humility to recognize that the gods—not always the doctors—play a very big role in who gets what disease, when, and whether or not the patients will get better. Under today's reimbursement schemes, thinkers are paid less than doers. As one family practitioner put it, this is one of "the errors of traditional health care, namely paying more for such as cutting, injecting, and imaging, than thinking."[7]

Medicare has a reimbursement schedule that's based on a system of what are called RVUs or relative value units, which is designed to characterize the work intensity of the *things doctors do* so as to prorate payments. The things with the highest relative values include heart, liver and lung transplantation; intracranial blood vessel repair; hand reimplantation; and pancreas and esophagus removal. All of these procedures have relative values greater than 50, while the essential day-to-day activities of health care like office consultation, subsequent hospital care and emergency department visit are valued at around 1. Put simply, a given hour of the higher-valued activity is, under the Medicare payment scheme, 50 times more valuable than an hour of what might well be preventive care.

The Medicare valuation system was devised largely by a group of physicians, and while one may quibble, it's a system that has stood the test of time and has adapted as new procedures have been developed. The highest-valued activities are the medical *tours de force*, procedures developed by doctors and procedures that only doctors will ever perform. No other provider group is competing to do those procedures that will remain the responsibility of highly motivated, highly trained, Extrovert/Thinker doctors. But there's a whole lot of competition at the lower end of the value scale.

Optometrists compete with ophthalmologists, and nurse midwives, with obstetricians. Nurse anesthetist organizations portray their members as just as good as, but less expensive than, physician anesthesiologists. The American Association of Nurse Anesthetists recently adopted a strategic plan requiring all of their newly credentialed nurses to become "Doctors of Nurse Anesthesia Practice."[8] And while the patient of the future will be wheeled off to the operating room by an anesthesia doctor, they'll have no idea, unless they ask, whether their provider is a doctor-doctor or a nurse-doctor.

Nurse practitioners, too, are moving to mandatory "doctoral preparation." The American Association of Nurse Practitioners has prepared their own strategic "roadmap" by which it will advance the "terminal degree for advanced practice nursing from the Master's to the Doctor of Nursing Practice (DNP) by the year 2015."[9] As we'll see in the next chapter, nurse practitioners can now be found in many medical offices, working side by side with doctors as well as in stand-alone urgent care centers and drugstore walk-in clinics.

The boundaries that once separated nurse from physician, primary care doctor from specialist, and internist from surgeon are being breached. Nurses are becoming doctors, cardiologists are doing what used to be cardiac surgery, gastroenterologists are operating with endoscopes, and radiation oncologists use sophisticated forms of radiation like proton beam therapy to compete with urologists for prostate cancer business.

We're in a cutthroat era of medical evolution. Change will be fast-paced. Individuals or specialties that are slow to adapt will fall behind. There will be many more Bryan Scherrs who drop out of the herd—specialists who become too slow or too fat or lose their teeth and fall prey to the ever-circling predators. Successful survivors may find safety in numbers, forming large multi-specialty groups. Medicine is indeed entering its own brave new world.

CHAPTER 15

MOTHER'S DAY

Like many families, our local members gather on Mother's Day to honor the women we married and the women who raised us. Mother's Day is celebrated around the world in many forms. In Ireland and the United Kingdom, for example, it's called Mothering Sunday and typically occurs in the spring of the year. Some date the roots of this holiday to ancient Greek or Roman customs honoring goddess mothers. Flowers are often given as gifts, and the feted mothers are often urged to take a day of rest while their spouses and children handle the cooking as best they can, which makes for some fascinating culinary adventures.

On one recent Mothering Day Sunday, my brother Chris volunteered to host and cook. My youngest sibling stayed largely within his comfort zone—he doesn't watch a lot of the Food Network—whisking up some mostly mashed potatoes, a green salad and a delightful variety of grilled chicken pieces: skinless-boned breasts, skinless thighs with bones, and skinned legs. But he did make one daring and unexpected additional course—one that doesn't usually accompany the traditional American chicken dinner.

Ever thoughtful, my mother, who was to be feted that night, had acquired some crisp "baby" asparagus spears, straight from a local farmers' market; and my brother, who didn't have a lot of experience with fresh asparagus but wanted to acknowledge the gesture, knew that the classic approach to this vegetable involved immersion in hot water. So he set a pot of same on the stove and heated it to a full rolling boil.

By this time, the women of mothering age had been shooed out of the kitchen. My sib was therefore unsupervised for a period and, like most men, not willing to seek direction. He plopped the baby asparagus spears into the boiling water and headed out the back door to attend to the chicken, which was, at that very moment, on fire on the grill. By the time he got back to the vegetables, they had already passed through most of the several stages of asparagus death and dying—from too chewy to crisp to soggy and then, finally, to a dark green, flaccid, paste-like mush.

Chris is very attentive to Mom. He's the baby boy, after all. He knew he had to serve this costly and specially delivered favorite of my mother's to the rest of us, because she had brought it to him as a gift. But now he realized he needed a Plan B. His eyes darted desperately around the kitchen, pausing briefly on peeled potato skins, dirty pots and pans, spilled milk, the toaster, the blender and the microwave. He looked everywhere, in fact, except at the soggy, still-steaming vegetable, which was now draining in a colander. From this, he averted his eyes.

Then, as if a light bulb had clicked on, his head swiveled slowly back to the two electrical appliances with which he was most comfortable. He'd definitely used the microwave to good effect before, on prefabricated meals specifically designed for that appliance, and he understood how to use it. While the gas stove and the grill had let him down before, the microwave had always been a good friend. But even he knew that the microwave was unlikely to bail him out of this particular problem with what were already overcooked vegetables. On the other hand, the blender—hmmm!

This explains why I wasn't really paying enough attention at dinner a bit later when my wife, Beth, started a story about her recent attempt to get our three kids vaccinated for swine flu. I was preoccupied with his "asparagus soup," which consisted of a finely blended mix of two-percent milk, onions, garlic powder and overcooked asparagus. This concoction was served to all of us at room temperature while my wife was entertaining the other mothers with a story involving her frustrations with a recent medical interaction—a topic so universally understood and safe, like the weather, that it can be safely trotted out in almost any venue.

In this particular instance, while my mouth, brain and stomach were preoccupied with the unusual culinary treat in my mouth, my ears vaguely registered the fact that my wife was saying that she had recently taken the kids to get their vaccinations at a MinuteClinic. I thought to myself: "Wait!

What? Really? I didn't know about this! Aren't they those drugstore doctors!? In fact, come to think of it, *are* they even doctors!? I think they're actually nurses! Like my wife!... Oh."

Now, I was in a quandary. As far as I was concerned, these MinuteClinic people are what many of my physician brethren would identify as "The Enemy." Some of my doctor friends would probably even say that they're nurses just masquerading as doctors. And, as I verified later, the MinuteClinic website does indeed feature an attractive woman smiling out of the screen with a stethoscope draped over the shoulder of her long, doctor-like, white coat. But the woman is actually and explicitly either a "master's prepared nurse practitioner" or a "physician assistant," according to the site's promotional materials. MinuteClinic is very clear that these are qualified, licensed, certificated and experienced practitioners.

It took me a long time to dispose of the spoonful of asparagus and milk in my mouth (I didn't end up swallowing it for a variety of reasons), and it was probably just as well that I couldn't blurt out my first thoughts. My wife went on to explain that she had gone to MinuteClinic because she couldn't deal with the concept of waiting two hours or more to get the kids their shots. And every other adult at the table, except me, was already nodding his or her head vigorously. "Yes!" "Yes!" They, *too,* had had it with the long waits in doctor's offices and thought the MinuteClinic idea was *perfect* for this kind of thing.

Had I actually said what was on the tip of my tongue, which was bathed in asparagus soup, about "Nurses!" and "Costumes!" and "Idiotic...," Mother's Day might not have ended very amicably. To be fair, *I* don't really understand how a doctor can already be two hours behind schedule by 10 o'clock in the morning, as is often the case in my own visits to my colleagues. I, too, sit there and stew just like almost everyone else in the waiting area.

It's pretty ironic that my wife and I, who, as a nurse practitioner and doctor, respectively, are the ultimate medical insiders, would ever need to resort to something like the MinuteClinic to get flu shots for the kids. But that's why the company's business model makes so much sense and why CVS bought what was originally called QuickMedx in 2006. It has subsequently installed these nurse-run clinics in many of its stores around the country.

QuickMedx was originally founded in 1999 after a casual watercooler conversation among its founders, who happened to be meeting to talk about another medical startup. They got diverted into a discussion about medical waiting areas after one of them started in on the hassle he had just gone through in a clinic the night before.

Rick Krieger was complaining about having waited several hours to get a simple rapid strep test for his son's sore throat at an urgent care center in Minneapolis. It turned out that another guy at the cooler, QuickMedx cofounder Steve Pontius, had just been through a similar experience a couple of weeks earlier with his own five-year-old son, who'd had an earache. Both had taken their kids to the doctor with what they recognized was a fairly straightforward and common medical condition, but one that required a test or a prescription to handle, and both had waited hours. The solution to each kid's problem required the intervention of a licensed medical professional just to prescribe a test or antibiotic. Recognizing a niche, Pontius, Krieger and a third partner quickly sketched up a business plan for a delivery model in which a limited slate of services was offered at a flat rate of $35 per encounter. The first QuickMedx clinics opened within a year.

QuickMedx originally targeted the individual patient, but that approach proved to be problematic. Too few patients used the service, and profit margins were too slim. The company's initial returns didn't meet the founders' projections, so they left the company by 2002. QuickMedx then became MinuteClinic, and a new management team took over with a slightly different business model. Rather than targeting individual walk-in patients, the new CEO, Linda Hall Whitman, focused on large insurers and employers that reimbursed their employees directly for care. This approach proved much more successful.

The larger insurance and corporate entities incented their employees to use MinuteClinic's relatively inexpensive and convenient services by techniques like reducing co-payments for a visit and emphasizing the convenience of the service. This implicit endorsement by their employer helped, and within two years, MinuteClinic had treated almost 50,000 patients. Today, the company advertises over 6 million visits in sites all over the country. Hosting facilities include CVS pharmacies, grocery stores, and corporate and governmental office buildings.

My wife's visit to our local CVS-based MinuteClinic typifies most such encounters. She needed seasonal flu shots for our three boys, and she knew from long years of experience with our pediatric practice that any attempt to engage in anything other than a scheduled appointment less than six months in advance would involve entering into what sounds like a bullfight. As she describes the process, step one is the initial call to the office, which is fielded by a receptionist. The clinic's receptionists are all highly skilled secretarial *picadors,* who deftly engage in what bullfighting aficionados would call the *tercio de varas*—the first portion of the highly ritualized contest between a mother and the pediatrician's office.

Picadors ride in pairs on horses protected from the bull's horns with mattress-like armor. A picador carries a lance, and he has three main jobs. The first is to pierce the muscles at the back of the bull's neck and thereby straighten its charge. The bull's attempts to gore and lift the padded horse are exhausting. After a few go-rounds with a mounted picador, even a strong bull fatigues, which is the picador's second task. It's not good to have a frisky bull when the matador enters the ring. And the third, critical role of the picador is to lower the bull's head by damaging its neck muscles in preparation for the next stage. A skilled picador leaves the bull still energetic but less willing to toss its head about during its subsequent confrontation with the matador. Like picadors, a pediatrician's secretarial staff, if good, leaves even the most anxious and energetic parent head down and fatigued in preparation for the next layer of pediatric defense.

The second third of a traditional bullfight, the *tercio de banderillas,* features *banderilleros.* The job of these apprentice matadors is to place sharp, decorative, barbed sticks into the neck or shoulders to anger and reinvigorate the bull, who may have become *too* fatigued or even apathetic during his encounter with the *picadors.* There are three *banderilleros,* which is fitting, because it typically takes at least three phone calls, involving several different nurses, before the by-now very bullish parent is sufficiently exhausted and agitated to finally engage with the pediatrician.

This third, concluding, *tercio*—the *tercio de muerte*—is the one from which a highly skilled matador may emerge with flowers or, perhaps, with the ear or tail of the now-*muerte* bull. To be fair to the sport, a real bull who has performed particularly well in the ring may, sometimes, be rewarded as well. When a bullfighting arena's crowd awards an *indulto* to a particularly courageous bull, his life is spared and he is returned to the ranch to live out the remainder of his life as a stud. Sadly, too few parents emerge from the pediatrician encounter with an *indulto.*

Rick Krieger and Steve Pontius both passed through their *tercios* while waiting with sick kids in a clinic, which led them to create QuickMedx. And while the division of labor in my household has sheltered me from most of these pediatric encounters, I *have* experienced the roll-down effects when defusing my wife after a couple of *tercios* at our Kid's Kare Klinik. Fortunately, she decided to try something new this year during flu season and went to MinuteClinic instead, only five minutes down the road. It requires no appointment, thereby bypassing the *picadors*. There is no prescreening by *banderilleros*. And there is no pediatrician *matador* in residence.

The MinuteClinic is more like a beauty salon. There's a menu of services. The client chooses the desired service, gets it and leaves. My wife selected three seasonal flu shots at $30 a pop, the kids got them and she left ten minutes later. Completely painless, except for the kids of course, and my wife was able to buy hair and dental products while they were getting stuck.

MinuteClinic offers a menu of services under the heading "minor illness exam" for about $60 or a co-payment with the patient's insurance company. This includes the diagnosis and management of things like flu symptoms, sore throat or earache, nasal congestion and urinary tract infections. "Minor injuries" such as blisters, burns, bug bites, splinters and lacerations are priced similarly. Covered "skin conditions" include cold and canker sores, chicken pox, scabies and shingles. MinuteClinic can also screen for high blood pressure ($30), diabetes ($40) and asthma ($95). The practitioners will perform a variety of specialty examinations for camp, school, college or sports that cost between $30 and $40. Pregnancy testing is $50. Ear-wax removal, oddly, is a little bit of a bargain, costing $3 less than most other procedures. Almost every service costs less than $100.

After my wife's Mother's Day confession, I decided to visit the nearest MinuteClinic to get a visual and to do an on-site investigation. They were my kids *too,* after all! Located in our nearby CVS, the clinic is unobtrusively integrated into the back of the store and conveniently positioned right next to the pharmacy. Wearing dark glasses so no acquaintance would recognize me during my research as a potential patient of this doctor-less medical facility, I shopped for a few things I didn't really need—chewing gum, a magazine—while scoping out the scene. As I browsed, I slowly worked my way back toward the clinic area, which has a big MinuteClinic logo on the wall. There were two exam-room doors straddling a large kiosk on which a display screen listed services and prices in a big, boldly colored, sans-serif font.

A tanned, long-haired, older man, wearing jeans that were cinched up above his navel and a pinkie ring was using a stylus to enter personal information and his medical complaints onto a touch screen. A woman and a young girl sat further down the wall in one of several sturdy chairs scattered in front of the exam rooms. The man seemed preoccupied by his task, peering a little closer at the screen every now and then as if puzzled by a prompt. Then he looked around quickly as if to make sure no one was watching over his shoulder. He, too, was wearing dark glasses but seemed suspicious of mine.

Both of the exam-room doors were shut. One read, "Closed for the day," and displayed a list of clinic hours. The other had a sign saying, "Clinician is with Patient, Please Wait." I decided to sit down in a chair to continue my investigation while I pretended to browse the internet on my cell phone, which was difficult with polarized dark glasses. I waited while the man finished logging in, after which he sat down in a chair a couple of seats away from me, glancing over nervously in my direction every couple of minutes.

Finally, partly to put him at ease, I hopped up to engage with the terminal. The home page showed the list of the people ahead of me in the queue with an approximate wait time and then prompted me for personal information. Had I been to MinuteClinic before? What service was I looking to purchase? I entered a fictitious patient name with "aches and pains all over" and moved on when a new client walked up. So far, so good, since I had no intention of following through with an actual visit.

Then I retreated to a more remote vantage point, because it was getting crowded and I wanted to see what the clinician and the client looked like. It took about 15 minutes for the transaction that was already underway, during which I spent a lot of time perusing the extensive array of eye lubricants and contact lens management systems sold by the store. I thought this seemed like a good way to justify the dark glasses, although I don't think I fooled either the long-haired guy or the store security system. The first finally left before he was seen, darting a nervous look back over his shoulder at me as he exited the store, and there were several passes by store employees who looked at me suspiciously.

Eventually, the exam-room door opened and a middle-aged guy emerged with what appeared to be his son. Both looked happy, and they proceeded directly to the pharmacy counter, where they seemed to be expected. The pharmacist handed over a vial of pills, and after the transaction was complete, the man and boy left. The whole process took a minute or two. A woman came out of the exam room at the same time and waved as they walked by. She looked like she had walked right out of a Norman Rockwell magazine cover.

Fiftyish, slightly overweight, with reading glasses on a leash, she wore a starched white coat with a MinuteClinic logo over its breast pocket holding a couple of pens. You could see that the pocket got a lot of use, because she obviously had put the pen away a couple of times before capping the tip. A stethoscope was draped over her shoulder. She looked motherly and competent.

She saw the young girl sitting with her mother, made a big fuss over her dress—completely and immediately disarming the child—and the smiling mother, her daughter and the "well-qualified MinuteClinic professional" disappeared back into the room. All in all, it looked like a pretty efficient, slick operation and, with the exception of the guy in front of me in line, I'd already seen a couple of satisfied customers.

MinuteClinics are designed to run lean. The patient enters relevant information into the clinic's electronic medical record software via a touch screen while waiting to be seen. The clinician then follows a series of logic-driven questions once she's in the room with the patient. The company compares this to a pre-flight checklist, and the logic is designed to arrive at a diagnosis and a focused treatment plan. Most importantly from a liability standpoint, the computer's software, like that of the avatar described in a previous chapter, is designed to determine whether or not the client's problem lies within a suite of common, readily characterized illnesses and, if so, to recommend a treatment course that's consistent with nationally accepted clinical practices. These best-practice algorithms are drawn from professional societies like the American Academy of Family Physicians, the American Academy of Pediatricians and the Institute for Clinical Systems Improvement. MinuteClinic also makes it very clear that they know when to refer a patient for issues that fall outside their defined scope of engagement.

MinuteClinic isn't the only company to offer fast, appointment-free medical care. While this company is owned by CVS, Walgreens owns Take Care Clinics, which use essentially the same model. A third company, The Little Clinic, has positioned *its* retail medical "storefronts" in supermarkets in several states and was recently acquired by Kroger, a large grocery retailer.

Walmart and Target also have developed retail health clinics, and FastCare and RediClinic are other brands.

Almost 90 percent of retail medical clinic visits are for one of ten common conditions that would otherwise require a visit to a primary care physician or emergency room. A typical visit requires no appointment and takes 15 to 20 minutes. The transaction costs one-third less than an urgent care appointment and three-quarters less than an emergency department evaluation. And because most of these visits are goal oriented, the patient typically leaves with a solution and is therefore a satisfied customer who will probably return. Rick Krieger had waited several hours with his son when his goal was to get a strep test that took seconds, while his partner Steve Pontius had needed a prescription for his son's earache. Like many medical transactions, these represent a set of clear-cut, uncomplicated problems that *could be* addressed in a brief encounter but typically *aren't* at traditional medical facilities because of the tremendous inefficiencies of the latter in delivering sub-acute care.

Harvard Business School Professor Clayton Christiansen and Dr. Jason Hwang co-authored a 2009 book entitled *The Innovator's Prescription: A Disruptive Solution for Healthcare.* They suggest three alternative approaches that business executives might adopt to reduce health-care costs to their companies. The first is to encourage their employees to use health-care retailers like MinuteClinic, the second is the formation of partnerships with integrated health systems like Kaiser Permanente, and the third is to set up their own clinics based on a retail model. Christiansen is best known for his studies of innovation, in particular, disruptive innovations—ones that enter a market at a relatively low cost and with modest goals but eventually go on to transform that market entirely.

The first personal computers, digital cameras and firearms, for example, were not perceived to be competitive with (refrigerator-sized) "minicomputers," traditional cameras or longbows, respectively, when they first became available. But as these products evolved, they became increasingly functional and eventually supplanted their predecessors. Through progressive innovation and performance improvements, today's "microcomputers" (PCs), digital cameras, guns and desktop printers have completely displaced the technologies they were originally developed to mimic. The imitators eventually became far more functional and less expensive than the originals. And it's not just products that can disrupt. Innovative services can disrupt the same way. Discount retailers like Walmart, Kmart and Target started with a limited scope in the 1960s but went on to disrupt and displace full-service department stores.

Christiansen and Hwang, the latter a former Kaiser Permanente physician and Harvard Business School graduate, believe that the retail medical care model exemplified by MinuteClinic represents a similarly disruptive innovation that will, with time, have a revolutionary effect on traditional medical care. And there is some reason to believe that they may be correct. While in 2006 there were only 200 American retail medical clinics, largely clustered in a few geographic areas such as the Great Lakes region of the United States, today there are over a thousand in 40 of the 50 states and dozens of companies competing for patients. Evidently the mothers at my brother's house on Mother's Day aren't the only ones who see value in hassle-free medical care.

Christiansen and Hwang, as well as a growing number of companies, believe that retail medical care represents an efficient, effective alternative to the traditional, oftentimes dysfunctional, alternative. Several seemingly unrelated trends suggest that there is good reason to pay attention to the evolution of retail medicine. Rising deductibles, for example, are likely to make consumers more conscious of the price differential between an emergency department visit, with the invariably lengthy wait, versus a convenient, much less expensive visit to a retail medical facility. As much as 20 percent of routine primary care visits are for diagnoses that fall within the limited number of conditions on which retail clinics concentrate. This includes the evaluation of flu-like syndromes and minor skin conditions as well as routine medical evaluations.

Handled properly by retail providers, a significant volume of business could get siphoned away from primary care physicians, urgent care centers and emergency rooms. And as with many disruptive innovations, there is a niche for the innovator's entry into a market that doesn't appear, at least at the outset, to present a big threat to the incumbent. Because of the typically low reimbursement rate for care provided to patients with these issues, most physicians don't see the loss of these sorts of patient visits as a problem. The problem, however, as with all disruptive innovations, is mission creep.

Retail medical care is already showing signs that it wants to grow beyond its modest initial scope. Whereas the company initially confined itself to the management of acute conditions and vaccines, it added cholesterol, blood pressure and diabetes screenings in 2003 and now provides ongoing monitoring of those conditions as well as asthma. Although the American Academy of Family Physicians was an ally at one point, co-signing explicit formal relationships with several retail health providers, it saw enough of an evolving threat that it issued the following statement in 2010:

> The American Academy of Family Physicians (AAFP) opposes the expansion of the scope of services of Retail Health Clinics and, in particular, the management of chronic medical conditions in this setting. The AAFP is committed to the development of a health care system based on strong, team based patient centered primary care defined as first contact, comprehensive, coordinated and continuing care for all persons and believe that the RHC model of care further fragments health care.[1]

This alteration of policy was prompted in part by the explicitly stated plans of some retail medical companies to move forward into chronic disease management.

Digital cameras were initially used only for a limited set of applications because their quality was poor, but they were inexpensive and served a niche. Similarly, desktop printers didn't initially appear to threaten traditional offset printers as they allowed home users to perform certain tasks readily and cheaply. Downloadable single songs didn't appear to threaten the CD or DVD industries at first, either, but the subsequent success of online retailers, such as iTunes, that sold one song at a time at a discount, speaks for itself.

Medicine, too, has plenty of examples of innovations from within that have disrupted traditional treatments or service models. For example, coronary balloon angioplasty was initially used only for a very limited subset of patients with coronary narrowings or blockages and therefore didn't appear at first to represent a threat to cardiac surgeons. But, as we've seen, subsequent innovations, such as improved catheters, stents and techniques, eventually led to the emergence of a whole new sub-specialty. Just like Kodak and Digital Equipment Corporation—two once-proud industry leaders—once-busy thoracic surgeons, who thrived on the then-lucrative practice of cardiac bypass surgery, are now out of work or in an entirely different line of medicine. And coronary lesions are now being treated pharmacologically with statin-class drugs, which may, in turn, eventually eliminate the disease and the need for interventional cardiologists altogether.

According to Christiansen, there are typically three enablers that work conjointly in disruptive innovations: (1) a simplifying technology, (2) a business-model innovation and (3) what he calls a *disruptive value network*. Alone, any of the three can advance an industry along a predictable, evolutionary trajectory, but, when they all occur at the same time, the synergy can transform an industry very rapidly. An easy-to-understand example of a simplifying technology is the instant, point-and-click camera (and, depending on the era, that might mean the Kodak Brownie, the Polaroid or Apple's QuickTake digital camera), which converted a once-complicated, expert-only photographic process to one that anyone could accomplish with the press of a finger. New business models abound exemplifying the second enabler for disruption. FedEx guaranteed overnight delivery, and iTunes sold single songs. These are two widely cited examples in which the new business model differed radically from its predecessors.

Finally, by *disruptive value network,* Christiansen is referring to the establishment of a new process by which a product or service is delivered to the consumer. The online iTunes store, for example, delivers a single song, or an entire "album," directly to the consumer. By so doing, Apple not only provided a product directly to the consumer; it also eliminated the costs associated with the predecessor delivery network, which included CD and DVD manufacturers, CD and DVD hardware manufacturers and the stores that sold those CDs and DVDs. The new, disruptive value network delivers music directly, cheaply and efficiently to the consumer with a simple-to-use menu and transparent pricing structure. If this sounds familiar, it should, because these attributes also characterize the interface between the consumer and the retail medical clinic.

So how do retail medical clinics size up as potential innovative disruptors of traditional care models? What, for example, is the simplifying technology Christiansen says is required? As with many disrupters, retail medicine has focused to date on the low end of the market, addressing simple, high-volume diagnoses that can be readily described in an electronic algorithm and for which there are tangible solutions—think earache and antibiotics. The simplifying technology is the uncomplicated decision-support software that the providers and patients use to arrive at a diagnosis and treatment plan.

Using a child with a sore throat as an example, like Rick Krieger's son, let's imagine what might happen in a retail medical clinic. Depending on the child's age, the patient, or parent, first enters some basic information at the kiosk's electronic front end, providing the nurse practitioner with a starting point. She can then go on to ask a series of directed questions guided by the decision-support software built into the clinic's electronic medical record. At some time in the process, she may come to a decision-branch point that suggests she should refer the patient to a higher level of care. If, for example, the child has a stiff neck along with the sore throat, meningitis becomes a possibility and he belongs in an emergency ward.

If, on the other hand, everything is consistent with an uncomplicated viral or bacterial sore throat, the next step is to determine whether or not antibiotics are warranted. What's needed then is the rapid strep test that Krieger was seeking when he went to the clinic only to wait hours for it. The nurse practitioner in the retail clinic can perform this test in minutes and, if it's positive, prescribe antibiotics on the spot. As a result, a process that might once have been much more subjective—before we had the rapid strep test—and best performed by an expert pediatrician can now be codified and objectified into a computer-driven process and quickly delivered in a simplified fashion. Similarly, while a simple landscape photograph might once have required the services of an expert photographer to determine the right combination of lighting, camera settings and film to get good results, today's digital cameras are equipped with computer chips that do all of this automatically and instantaneously.

What about Christiansen's new-business-model requirement? Retail medical care unequivocally represents a new approach with its convenient location and pricing arrangements. Instead of requiring the customer, the patient in this case, to come to a hospital's facilities, adhere to its rules of engagement and endure its lengthy wait times, retail medical care is available in the places where the client shops or works and offers a shopping list of services. That's why banks have put branches in supermarkets.

Disruptive value networks, Christiansen's third requirement, are emerging as well. Some companies like Perdue Chicken and Miller Brewing have established on-site retail clinics, but most are located in pharmacies, supermarkets or discount retailers. Many health retailers have begun to establish relationships directly with insurers and pharmacies. The synergies are obvious: when I went to the retail clinic, the patient could pick up a prescription from the next window immediately after finishing the appointment with the provider. Contrast this with the hassles Steve Pontius encountered when he tried to get a prescription for his son with the earache.

These new value networks completely bypass the traditional physician provider and are much more efficient in delivering specific services to the patient. Today, if you want to buy a single from the latest *Britain's Got Talent* star, you need merely download from the online music vendor of your choice—no need to drive to the CD store or buy the whole album. Similarly, if all you need is a strep test for your son's sore throat and a prescription if warranted, you can drive a few minutes the nearest retail clinic and get it. Nearly instant gratification in both cases, but when it's your health, you want to get it right, right?

Emerging data about retail care suggests that these nurse-practitioner-run clinics do well with acute medical conditions. In an evaluation of nearly 60,000 cases of sore throat over a one-year period, 99 percent of the time, retail providers *did not* prescribe antibiotics to the two-thirds of the patients with a negative strep test. More importantly, they *did* prescribe appropriate antibiotics for the one-third with a positive test. Another study looking at the management of earache, sore throat and urinary tract infection at retail clinics showed that visits for these conditions cost substantially less compared to costs at doctor's offices, urgent care centers or emergency departments. The preventative care and quality scores were comparable at retail clinics, doctors' offices and urgent care centers but *lower* in emergency departments.

One of the key attributes of truly disruptive technologies is the fact that they enter the market at the bottom, where profit margins are small and the threat to the incumbent technology appears to be minimal. A cycle then ensues in which the disruptor innovates continuously, while the incumbent retreats up-market to retain higher-end and more profitable customers. The disruptor is driven to improve to enhance profits, while incumbents are fighting a series of retrenching battles until they are finally marginated into a small corner, or gone.

Christiansen notes three lessons from previous disruptive revolutions that he believes are relevant to health care. The first is that the technological underpinnings, the simplifiers, typically come from leading institutions, while the business model innovations come from the outside. Treatment algorithms for sore throat simplify medical care and are produced by professional societies, while Rick Krieger and his partners were business entrepreneurs when they started QuickMedx. A second lesson is that, to be effective, new value networks need to replace the old. To truly disrupt, retail medical clinics can't just be plugged into existing health networks; they must develop their own direct connections to employers, insurers and patients, bypassing hospitals and doctors.

The third lesson from previous successful revolutions of the past is that the energies of the incumbents are typically focused on improving the top end of their products. They complacently disparage seemingly simplistic technological innovations. Physicians who are trained to use the literature and their intelligence to diagnose and manage their patients find it inconceivable that a simple computer algorithm might perform as well as or better than they do. The threat, however, is very real.

I recently took a trip to Rochester, New York, to visit with some folks from Kodak Research, a laboratory that has produced over 20,000 patents since its inception in 1912. The trip from the airport to the organization's headquarters was striking. We passed mile after mile of huge, derelict, rusting buildings that were once part of the Kodak "you press the button and we do the rest" value network. The chemicals were brewed here, the film was manufactured here, pictures were developed here and those once unmistakable envelopes full of priceless "Kodak moments" were mailed from here. But the world moved on.

Despite the fact that many of the technologies fundamental to digital photography were invented by Kodak, this company, and many of the other film giants, failed to catch the digital wave in time. Kodak was delisted from the Dow Jones Industrial Average index on April 8, 2004, after three-quarters of a century as one of the top American companies. Curiously it was replaced in the index by American International Group, or AIG, which itself lasted only a few years before it was bailed out by the U.S. government in September 2008.

Even today, it seems inconceivable that medical care could undergo the same degree of fundamental transformation that the film industry did in such a short period of time. But one need only look to the music, publishing, telephone and retail industries to see examples of radical change in very short periods of time.

There is a war underway in medicine to take the once highly individualized and intuitive diagnostic and treatment algorithms that were unique to each physician and codify them into best practices. If you think of a medical best practice as just another widget, like a cell phone, a computer or a digital camera, you can imagine a process through which it evolves. Widgets, be they algorithms or products, can be subjected to ongoing study and continuous improvement, and best-practice widgets, once defined, can be tested for accuracy, efficacy and efficiency.

One can even imagine that through this evolutionary process, once-clunky best-practice widgets will eventually evolve to become as sleek and functional as today's smartphones and cameras. As they're formalized, they can get coded into software as decision-support tools that can be administered just as readily by a doctor, or a nurse practitioner, or even by the patient herself. It is entirely feasible that much of the cognitive work now performed by medical providers will eventually become so objective, precise and encodable that the doctor himself might become obsolete.

I don't personally believe this mechanized version of the future will ever become real because I think the most important element of the interaction between the doctor and the patient is fundamentally human. Medicine evolved from altruistic activities like mutual grooming and feeding that are common to species throughout the animal kingdom. However, we do need to find our way to some model of medical care that balances the opportunities provided by advances in medical technology with what's best for the patient. The patient-centered medical home, which we'll discuss in the next and last chapter of the book, looks to the past for ways to improve the future of medical care.

CHAPTER 16

OUT OF NETWORK

"Hi, Dr. Hanson!"

This greeting was shouted from a crowd of 8-year-olds who had just exited the classroom that I believed currently contained my own youngest child. The salutation was slightly unusual, since most kids that age don't engage with adults at all, if possible, or, at best, only when it is absolutely necessary. Of the ones who do, very few of them understand the fact that I am a physician and that we use a different honorific. As far as I'm concerned, even a "Hi, Mr. Hanson," with or without eye contact, rates an A.

I panned the crowd and identified the kid who had called out. He happened to be one of my very favorites—the youngest child in a family with whom we've shared school, sleepovers, athletic events—all of the village-based, child-rearing responsibilities. Jake is a really engaging little guy. He invariably says hello, is able to carry on a conversation consisting of full sentences and is engaging, funny and great with eye contact. So when I saw my little friend, I stopped looking for my son Cal, figuring he'd find me on his own. I asked Jake what was up, bumping fists with him. While we were talking, I went through the usual visual medical assessment I'd come to undertake routinely in any encounter with one of Jake's family. I usually turn this scanning function off when I'm with friends or family but not around Jake. Where was the injury this time, I asked myself?

Sure, every healthy kid has a cut, bruise or bandage periodically. But Jake and his siblings are *always* in treatment. I mean always. As soon as one kid enters physical therapy, another has surgery, typically for some orthopedic condition I've never heard of. This time, Jake had an elastic brace on his knee and was limping.

I formed my face into a look of concern and said, "What happened, bud?"

"Osgood-Schlatter," he answered brightly and immediately, pronouncing it correctly. And he gave me a knowing look.

He'd assumed, since I'm one of the limited number of doctors he knows personally, that I, too, knew exactly what that means. I imagine he figured that all doctors have exactly the same knowledge base. As it happened, I had heard of, but didn't exactly remember much about, Osgood-Schlatter disease, other than having a vague sense that it had something to do with pain, young people and joints. And I couldn't remember whether it is a transient problem, chronic and debilitating or, God forbid, terminal. For that matter, I wasn't sure whether it is communicable. So I was at a little bit of a loss as to how exactly to answer at first. If only he'd said, "I have a tibial tubercle apophyseal traction injury," I would have gotten it immediately.

I settled on the universal response I had learned in medical school for these sorts of situations in which one is expected to know the answer but doesn't—that being the "Knowing Nod." It seemed to work, because Jake went on to tell me that he'd be back off the disabled list in a couple of weeks.

Jake comes from what I have often mentally described as a *medical home,* where injuries and complaints are taken *very seriously,* and *investigated,* and *treated,* if at all possible. We all know families like this. Sometimes, it's the kids with injuries. In other variants, there are pill bottles on the Lazy Susan and in the spice drawer. In these households, antibiotics are dispensed with the vitamins, the parents use up their sick leave every year and the children are held home from school at the drop of a hat or the drip of a nose.

So you can imagine my surprise when I heard President Obama quoted during the run-up to the passage of the recent American health-care plan overhaul as saying, "I support the concept of a patient-centered medical home, and as part of my health care plan, I will encourage and provide appropriate payment for providers who implement the medical home model."[1] It wasn't immediately clear to me how this made sense.

Why would we want to encourage the kind of health-care consumerism indulged in by Jake's family? Wouldn't we be better off providing "appropriate payment for providers" like my father, who implemented what amounted to a "*No* Medicine in the Home Model." In our house, you had to be *very* sick to warrant medical attention. Dad once dismissed my complaints about a headache that turned into viral meningitis. Some would say that the "gate-keeper model" created to control health-care costs in the late 1990s was also a sort of "no medicine in the home (or elsewhere) model." But that paradigm presents challenging conflicts, as we've seen.

It turns out that President Obama was actually referring to a concept developed and espoused by modern primary care practitioners, some-what confusingly called the *patient-centered medical home*. The medical-home model was first described in the 1960s by the American Academy of Pediatrics and subsequently formalized and redefined by that organization in 1992. Its tenets were outlined in a joint position paper from the pediatric society, in partnership with the American Academy of Family Physicians, the American Osteopathic Association and the American College of Physicians. Combined, these organizations represent 330,000 American physicians. They support the establishment of patient-centered medical homes that are designed to foster partnerships between individual patients, their families, if appropriate, and a personal physician.

The principles of the medical home center on the establishment of an ongoing functional relationship between a patient and her doctor and are explicitly intended to counter the increasing fragmentation of patient care in our modern era of specialty medicine. The medical home's physician directs a team of practitioners that takes ongoing responsibility for the care of each patient, arranging and coordinating that care across time, space and specialties. The "whole-person orientation" of this relationship means that the patient's personal physician takes responsibility for direct provision of care when appropriate and "subcontracts" care when necessary to other— perhaps specialist—physicians or home-health providers. The medical-home personal physician remains actively engaged in, and coordinates through-out, all stages of care—and, indeed, throughout the patient's life—including acute, chronic and terminal care. This is the way medical care looked in Norman Rockwell's depictions of doctors on magazine covers in the 1920s, the way Marcus Welby managed his patients in the 1960s and the way my father handled his practice until his death on September 28, 1991.

My father's career began at a time when primary care providers could still provide all but the most complex care. During his 40-year practice, however, evolving specialties began to nibble away at the scope of problems that fell within his "comfort zone." Medical specialties became much more complex during that era, and *today's* typical primary care provider would look to a specialist for help in managing many of the problems that were once considered routine. While that may well be appropriate now, and best for the patient, neither is the case when it results in the fragmentation of care that occurs when a single patient's multiple medical problems are managed in an uncoordinated fashion.

According to the medical societies' position paper on the patient-centered medical homes, one of the key tenets of a medical home is that it ensures that "care is coordinated and/or integrated across all elements of the complex health care system (e.g. subspecialty care, hospitals, home health agencies, nursing homes) and the patient's community (e.g. family, public and private community-based services)."[2]

A close friend of mine whom I'll call "Nick Carson" was recently discharged from the hospital after a complicated brain operation. During the course of his hospitalization, he was treated by a number of hospital specialists, including a neurologist, an endocrinologist and a surgeon. He was originally referred to a neuro*surgeon* at the hospital; and the referral was made by his office-based primary care physician, who was not linked professionally with any of the hospital specialists, so the lines of communication among them were inefficient at best.

After surgery, Nick was transferred from the acute care facility to a rehabilitative hospital nearer his home, where he underwent intensive physical and mental therapy for a month. After his discharge from there to home, Nick had ongoing therapy on a more-or-less daily basis. His blood chemistries were carefully monitored with frequent laboratory tests, and his medications were adjusted by one of the hospital specialists based on the results of the tests. His medical problem was outside the expertise of his primary care doctor, so the drug management was being handled by the hospital's endocrinologist.

During his ongoing rehabilitation process, Nick and his wife ran into a very complicated problem that was identified by a blood test, but they were unable to get timely answers from the endocrinologist about the management of a critical medication. As a result, one night they were forced to go to the emergency room at a nearby local hospital for help. Unfortunately, Nick hadn't been seen at that hospital before, so he and his wife had to start from scratch in describing the issues, and it turned out that the emergency physician was unfamiliar with the management of the unusual endocrine problem for which they were seeking help. Consequently, they had to spend that night in the emergency department awaiting feedback from the unreachable endocrinologist, and it was only in the light of the following day, after multiple phone calls, that everything got sorted out.

Because the hospital they went to was "out of network," this whole, ultimately unnecessary, emergency visit wasn't covered by his insurance. Nick and Valerie now personally owed over a thousand dollars for this visit. And all this happened during a time when neither was able to work because of the complexity of Nick's illness. This is the kind of problem a medical home is intended to address.

In retrospect, many of the problems and inefficiencies my friend and his wife experienced throughout his recovery could have been eliminated had there been a single point of contact, the medical home, to which they could turn for coordination of his very complicated care. They should have been able, for example, to reach a provider from the medical home to get an answer about the management of that medication problem rather than make repeated calls to a hospital operator, who couldn't find an on-call endocrinologist. Advocates of the medical home, as well as many national health interest groups, envision a day when electronic medical records and efficient health-information exchange will allow a new doctor, like the emergency physician my friend saw, to have authorized access to a medical record when needed.

Recognizing the diversity of the population that flows through many medical facilities around the world, the medical-home model also speaks to the need for culturally and linguistically appropriate care. For example, I recently took a walk on Miami's South Beach and saw Orthodox Jews sunbathing side by side with sculpted South Americans and Europeans. The Orthodox Jews were fully clothed, while the others weren't. Miami's hospitals provide care for both populations; and this same diversity of nationalities, languages and comfort with body display is found in many hospitals. The medical-home model acknowledges the need for sensitivity to these cultural differences in the provision of medical care. Many hospitals today, for example, subscribe to telephonic translation services, providing a method for providers and patients speaking different languages to communicate effectively even in the absence of a physically present translator. And hospitals are increasingly sensitive to culturally specific issues. Some have even purchased hospital gowns designed specifically for Muslim men and women.

One of the aspects of medical homes that the Obama administration saw as fundamental to their success is an emphasis on objective measures of quality and safety. Medical homes rely on a planning process that includes the personal physician, the patient and her family in an explicit partnership. By the unambiguous use of the term *partnership,* professional societies who support the concept recognize the fact that each party brings an essential investment to the table in any medical relationship, ranging from simple health-maintenance visits to the complicated issues of elder or end-of-life care.

Medical-home care is guided by evidence-based medicine and clinical decision-support tools. Its physician providers agree to engage in continuous quality improvement as well as to permit monitoring of their performance and outcomes, practices that historically had been unwelcome by many doctors. On their part, medical-home patients are encouraged to take an active role in decision-making.

During the course of my own career, I've encountered a full spectrum of attitudes from patients and families about participation in the often-complicated decisions involved in the care of critically ill patients. There's the wide-eyed faith of the timid, elderly spouse who says, regarding the terminal care of his dying wife, "That's OK, doc, you decide. She trusted her doctors." At the other extreme, there's the roomful of hostile, slate-eyed family members, one of whom has a pencil and pad on hand and scribbles down every word I utter "for legal reasons." The latter are often patients and families who've had a prior bad interaction with a health-care professional and are understandably inclined to question almost everything uttered by a doctor.

There are obvious problems with both interactions, and the ideal case is one in which the doctor provides an open and full discussion of the issue at hand, the benefits and risks of treatments, the knowns and unknowns. The patient and, if appropriate, the family then have the right and indeed the responsibility to take an active role in decision making, accepting risks and unknowns in the process. The medical home is designed to foster these kinds of relationships.

Medical-home supporters and a growing percentage of providers believe information technology of one kind or another is essential to the success of these enterprises. Effective electronic information exchange through electronic health records, systems for entering physician orders and electronic prescribing will eventually knit into something that resembles today's internet; medical information will be updated continuously and automatically and available to authorized parties, wherever they be. Computerized decision-support tools will present evidence-based, best-practice recommendations to the provider or patient at the appropriate moment and in a useful fashion. Automated prompts, for example, can get built into these systems to remind the medical-home provider or patient that it's time for a flu shot, tetanus vaccine or mammogram.

My friends and family are very respectful of the line between my professional life and my personal life, but I do occasionally get a call from someone who's been pushed to the edge because they can't get through to their doctor with a question or can't even schedule an appointment for something relatively straightforward. They may want an answer to a question, some treatment advice or even a prescription. I usually "just say no" to the last because I am not in a position to make good decisions about best care when I don't know all of the relevant medical history, but I do go out of my way to help friends in their efforts to penetrate the pachydermatous skin of the health-care system.

Medical homes are designed to be thin-skinned, providing "enhanced access" for their patients. The model encompasses such concepts as open scheduling, expanded office hours and the development of new and enhanced methods for communication between the provider and the patient—presumably in contrast to the usual secretarial gauntlet. In the future, we are likely to see novel methods for patient-provider communication, ranging from electronic mail to text messaging on the one hand, and to live, interactive audio-video links on the other.

The final tenet of the medical-home statement of principles is that providers should be adequately compensated for the provision of these "value-added" services. Traditional medical payment schemes pay only for face-to-face time or procedures. For example, the requirements for the submission of a bill for critical care professional services to Medicare are very stringent. The standard code reads, "Critical care, evaluation and management of the critically ill or critically injured patient, first 30–74 minutes." The minute value represents the aggregated total time a physician spends in any calendar day providing care for the patient for whom the bill was submitted, but it "must be spent at the immediate bedside or elsewhere on the floor or unit as long as the physician is immediately available to the patient." Time spent updating the family in person or on the phone is not billable unless the patient is unable to speak for himself and the discussion is required to make decisions about treatment.

These explicit requirements are both reasonable and necessary, and are similar to the ones used to describe billable primary care encounters. But medical-home proponents envision an always-available medical provider, much like the old general practitioner. They believe that a patient like my friend Nick should never be hospitalized because someone can't reach his doctor—*but* they want doctors to be paid for their ready availability.

Professional societies advocating the medical-home model suggest that reimbursement should cover both the activities that do and those that do not fall within the confines of the traditional face-to-face visit. These include the coordination of care and communications with persons or agencies necessary to that coordination. They explicitly support payment schemes encouraging the adoption of information technologies for communication and remote monitoring. If, for example, as will soon become possible, a medical-home provider uses medical devices and video links to assess or communicate with a patient in his home, rather than in a face-to-face encounter, the societies feel that that care should be reimbursed. A medical home should also be responsive to the differing communication needs and technological sophistication of a heterogeneous mix of young and old or healthy and infirm patients.

Not surprisingly, the organizations representing the interests of primary care professionals believe that medical-home providers should benefit from good, cost-effective care by participating in any savings that result from a reduction in patient hospitalizations or by the demonstration of "measurable and continuous quality improvements." While this last bit sounds suspiciously like some of the cost-reduction mechanisms inherent in the now-discredited gatekeeper model of the 1990s, there is a key difference, one that should make it much more palatable to all parties. In the medical-home model, the physician steers, but the patient chooses.

The 1990s Clinton-era, American-managed-care gatekeeper model was introduced by health maintenance organizations like Kaiser Permanente. The patient's gatekeeping physician had to approve all referrals to a specialist as well as diagnostic studies and procedures. And the HMOs put the patient's personal physician at risk financially for the overall costs of patient management; so physicians who limited care in that model were rewarded financially. Unfortunately, the best gatekeepers ended up incurring the wrath of both the patients who wanted access to specialists *and* the specialists who wanted referrals of patients. Good gatekeeping could also be bad medicine, and gatekeepers were still at risk for malpractice claims. If, by attempting to manage a problem falling outside of his competence or comfort zone, a primary care gatekeeper 'injured' a patient, he could be sued either for "failure to diagnose" or for "failure to refer."

In contrast to this older managed-care model, the personal physician in the medical home acts as the *coordinator* of care rather than as a *gatekeeper*. She has access to a comprehensive picture of the patient's medical issues via an electronic medical record, and she is able to facilitate the provision of information to needed specialists and to thoughtfully coordinate care. The patient gets to select a personal physician and actively participates in the decision to see a specialist or undergo a procedure.

Five percent of Medicaid beneficiaries account for about 50 percent of its expenditures, and the typical patient has multiple chronic conditions. In fact, 80 percent of Medicaid recipients have three or more medical conditions, such as diabetes, asthma or hypertension; and 60 percent have *five* or more of these costly, complicated, chronic medical problems. Some experts estimate that the care of the subset of patients with multiple chronic conditions account for 75 percent of *total* health-care spending. The care of complicated patients is not merely a problem of the poor or underinsured; it cuts across all socioeconomic groups.

I have several older relatives with more than one chronic condition. One of my favorites is Uncle Fred. He's on a blood thinner because he's had a heart valve replacement. He's also had a knee replacement for an old football-related injury, a stroke that left him speechless for a period, a bulging disk with sciatica and prostate cancer. He's also a "snowbird," spending part of his winters in the South and summers in the Northeast. Uncle Fred likes to travel and play golf. And he has lots of doctors. He has local doctors for day-to-day care near his home. There's another set of doctors in the big city, a two-hour drive away, who are on special teams reserved for more complicated care. There are also taxi-squad doctors in the South. They only get called in when he's down there during the winter and develops an unexpected medical problem.

It seems like Fred has to see at least one doctor or another almost weekly, as does his wife, Dolly. Both of them spend a lot of time shuttling back and forth between family, their doctors and their friends. The biggest problem seems to be that there is little to no coordination among their various doctors, the medical records and scheduled diagnostic and therapeutic activities. At best, the cardiologist may copy the internist on a letter or Fred might carry a DVD with his x-ray studies back and forth from one physician to another. All of these doctors currently act as independent agents; there is no real incentive for them to communicate amongst themselves or for any one of them to act as a central coordinator. The medical-home model is designed to remedy the problems inherent in Uncle Fred and Aunt Dolly's nomadic medical wanderings.

In a typical Medicaid population, patients bounce from one appointment to another, tests are repeated unnecessarily, drugs may be prescribed for one condition that exacerbate another and the provider of last—and too often, most frequent—resort is the emergency department. Two of the oldest and most mature medical-home programs in the United States are run by North Carolina's Medicaid managed-care program.

The first small pilot of what eventually developed into the first medical home started in 1988. North Carolina's Medicaid agency negotiated an arrangement with two medical practices guaranteeing reasonable reimbursement for regular visits plus an extra "case management" fee amounting to around $30 per patient per year. In return for this supplemental payment, the practices took on responsibility for coordinating the care of the covered patients. In other words, the doctors agreed to do what a general practitioner would have done routinely a generation or so ago: to act as the point of first contact for the complicated patients who typify many Medicaid populations. This arrangement proved to be so popular with its participant patients and doctors and so cost-effective that the state decided to expand its investment in this new model. The vast majority of the state's Medicaid patients are now enrolled in medical-home programs.

The first pilot program was developed by the North Carolina Office of Rural Health in conjunction with the Kate B. Reynolds Charitable Trust, one of the state's largest altruistic funds. Wilson County is a small rural county, and two large multispecialty practices serviced the majority of the county's Medicaid patients in 1988. The funding from the Reynolds Charitable Trust was entirely consistent with its mission supporting health and wellness in

North Carolina's citizens. While the fund has its roots in tobacco (Kate Bittig was married to William Neal Reynolds, the then-chair of the R. J. Reynolds tobacco company), it was endowed in 1947, long before tobacco money acquired its current taint.

As a member of one of North Carolina's leading families, Kate Reynolds lived in luxury on the Tanglewood Estate, a thousand-acre spread where the family raised racehorses. Now better known as Tanglewood Gardens, the Reynolds's bequest transferred it to Forsyth County in 1951. Mrs. Reynolds had an abiding interest in the poor; during her lifetime, she established community hospitals and supported better wages for workers, affordable housing for women and good day care for children.

The Health Care Division of the Reynolds Trust now works explicitly to support the design of solutions that improve the quality of health for needy North Carolina residents through prevention as well as through treatments that are "creative, relevant, and useful in tackling today's challenges and preventing tomorrow's problems."[3] In 1988, the first medical home that was funded by the Trust met all of these requirements. The subsequent proliferation of the model in the state demonstrates the foresight of the trustees and is an outstanding example of the potential synergies between charitable contributions and governmental initiatives.

As a governmental agency, Medicaid acts as both an insurer and a regulator. Probably due to the latter role, it is typically viewed by physicians with a degree of distrust. But with strong and respected leadership, North Carolina Medicaid was able to forge bonds with local physicians in the 1990s in expanding the medical-home project across the state. A more or less organic, self-organizing partnership developed, involving individual practices, state medical societies and state government. The demonstration medical homes, which were initially designed solely to coordinate the medical care of indigent patients, "metastasized" throughout the state and eventually coalesced into an organic, integrated delivery network like some mythic part-private, part-government beast.

These original medical homes were intended to do three things: to enhance patients' access to primary care, to improve the coordination of that care and to reduce the reliance on emergency-department visits for basic medical problems like the cough, flu-like symptoms or back pain that bring many patients to the emergency room. But by achieving these simple goals, medical homes saved North Carolina a lot of money, so the state became more ambitious and grew the program. After trying several alternatives, Medicaid concluded that a regionalized (instead of centralized) management approach worked best.

Rather than imposing a traditional top-down hierarchy run from the state's capital in Raleigh, the state set up 14 networks for coordination from a regional level. Each had its own physician medical director, typically a well-regarded local practitioner who could work well with primary care physicians whom he knew personally. Recognizing that most small primary care practices, which typically consist of one or two physicians and a support staff, would be unable to coordinate the round-the-clock care of a cadre of Medicaid patients even with the medical-home subsidy, the networks identified all of the relevant support resources in a given region. They set up mechanisms to facilitate cooperation among the participants by arranging for cross-coverage among the small practices and by supporting nurse case managers who work with several practices at the same time.

The importance of a case manager, typically a registered nurse with good interpersonal skills, is amply clear from a vignette described in a profile about North Carolina's medical homes in *Governing* magazine.[4] The publication described a series of encounters between a primary care doctor and the mother of a 9-month-old boy with asthma. The doctor thought the child's repeated asthma flare-ups and the resulting trips to emergency rooms were probably due to dust around the house; dust mites are a typical offender in many allergic diseases. He suggested that Mom clean and vacuum as carefully as possible. But the asthma proved to be very difficult to treat, and the flare-ups continued regularly despite aggressive treatment. The mother and child lived in a trailer home in a rough part of town, and the doctor eventually concluded that the house was just not well kept. However, as the nurse case manager found when she visited, the trailer was spotless.

It turned out that the mother had been cleaning house every couple of days as the doctor had suggested, and she used lots of bleach. It also became apparent that the child's asthma reliably flared up every time a clean-up occurred while he was at home. The caustic fumes of the bleach were what provoked the wheezing. Once the mother stopped using as much bleach, the flare-ups stopped, as did the need for unplanned trips to the emergency room. By visiting the boy and his mother in their trailer, the medical-home case manager was better able recognize the real source of the problem, and thereby to manage medical care and secondarily to reduce costs. This same kind of story was repeated over and over again in one form or another as the medical-home model proliferated throughout North Carolina. The state has by now realized hundreds of millions of dollars of savings from its medical homes since 1988.

While the North Carolina system is a "network of networks" involving lots of otherwise-unconnected small practices, medical homes have also developed within established hospital networks, such as the Geisinger Health System in central Pennsylvania. It provides round-the-clock access to primary care doctors supplemented by nurse coordinators, case managers and home monitoring. Geisinger uses standard electronic records that are accessible to both practitioners and patients. Patients using these records can see their own labs, schedule visits online and communicate directly with their providers using email. The providers can send relevant information or reminders to patients.

In addition to developments like the patient-centered medical home, other major medical shifts have been occurring. Direct-to-consumer advertisement of prescription drugs was first permitted in the mid-1990s, and within a decade the pharmaceutical industry was spending billions to bring brand name products like Viagra, Nexium, Valtrex and Lunesta into the day-to-day conversations of the average man-on-the-street as well as into conversations between doctor and patient. Similarly, direct-to-consumer marketing on billboards and television has become a way for hospitals and professional societies to keep their medical specialists in the forefront of the minds of potential patients.

In the last 20 years, the veil between the patient and the previously occult world of medicine has been whisked aside. When my father began his practice, a new patient came to the doctor's office with very little information about medicine in general, much less about what might be wrong with him. In that era, my father represented a kind of high priest of medicine who knew the "Sacred Knowledge" and dispensed magical drugs.

Today, once-sacrosanct medical texts have been scanned by Google. Medical schools, professional societies and patient groups all have websites explaining diseases and treatment options. The *Merck* manual is even available as a cell-phone app. Drugs for the treatment of common and once-embarrassing medical problems, with their intended effects and unwanted side effects, are described in excruciating and often embarrassing detail in television commercials and print ads. And medical specialists who used to be hidden in the shadows behind the primary care doctors have thrown open their doors to welcome patients directly into their offices, promoting "brand awareness" with billboards, television advertisements and web outposts.

All of this new transparency about drugs and doctors is for the good in many ways, but many patients suffer from what my children call *too much information*. There's now *so* much information flooding out to the consumer that most don't know what to do with it and often tune it out. At the same time, despite the incessant hawking of medical wares of one sort or another, access to and navigation through the vast and complicated health-care system remains a huge problem.

Many, including primary care doctors and governmental advocates, believe that the medical-home model will remedy problems with access to and fragmentation of care, while avoiding those inherent in the physician-as-gatekeeper approach. Medical homes are a sort of "return to the future" for medicine, providing patients with the kind of service once commonly offered by general practitioners of my father's generation—for example, round-the-clock availability and comprehensive care. While these are patient-oriented benefits, many policy makers see the financial benefit of channeling medical interactions through the neck of a funnel—the medical home—as a way to gain greater control over the delivery of medical care.

The growing prominence of medical homes obviously tilts the balance of power between primary care providers and specialists—pushing the locus of control back toward the former. The American Academy of Pediatrics, the American Academy of Family Physicians, the American Osteopathic Association and the American College of Physicians all represent separate groups of physicians, but their constituencies are all primary care physicians. It is in their interests to support—and run—medical homes, particularly if they get paid an extra, per-patient management fee. Not surprisingly, the specialists have taken note, particularly since the money spent on medical homes will ultimately come from funds that would otherwise go to specialists.

Some specialty groups have argued that *their* disciplines can actually serve as a kind of medical home for patients with certain chronic conditions. Endocrinologists, for example, see many patients with diabetes and often act as primary care physicians for diabetics, and pulmonologists do so for patients with chronic lung diseases, such as emphysema or asthma.

Urologists have actually claimed to act as "principal care physicians" for patients with prostate cancer.

It remains to be seen whether the medical-home model will be widely successful and durable. At first, gatekeeping seemed like a good idea, but the model and its title proved to be unacceptable to various constituencies. Patients don't like "gates" or their keepers. By describing one's practice as a "medical home," on the other hand, particularly, a "patient-centered medical home," a pediatrician or internist is already off to a better start.

My father practiced during the transition from an era when specialists were used infrequently to one in which specialists proliferated. Their scope of practice expanded inexorably into management of the medical problems he once handled competently and comfortably. To be fair, this encroachment was invariably the function of the growth of information and techniques in the specialty. Cardiac catheterization, for example, hadn't even been invented when he began to practice in the 1950s, when "coronaries" were managed with what we doctors call *therapeutic nihilism*—our way of saying that "there's nothing to be done."

While my father's management of a heart attack might have amounted to what he called *masterful inactivity* in the 1960s, before the advent of what we now call interventional cardiology, a comparable patient today could develop symptoms, go to his local hospital, be flown from there by helicopter to a facility equipped for cardiac emergencies and undergo immediate catheterization and treatment on arrival—all of which might take no more than a few hours. By the end of his career, my father came to be recognized for his ability to coordinate the care of his patients in a hospital full of specialists. He was a doctor's doctor, respected by his peers and patients for his ability to provide the human face to an increasingly fragmented and high-tech health-care delivery system.

Because our careers and professions overlapped, unlike too many of today's fathers and sons, I had the good fortune to be able to work side by side with him for a few years, just as father-and-son farmers or craftsmen have done in the past. I covered his medical practice occasionally when he was away, which was the source of a deep, mutual, quiet satisfaction. We were able to use this common ground to communicate the things that fathers and sons often find difficult to put into words. On my part, this was: "I admire you and try to be like you." On his, I think, it was: "You've grown up to be someone I trust to take up this work that I've handled alone for these many years." These same unspoken conversations have occurred over the centuries in farm fields, factories and mines, but, one suspects, less so in today's rapidly changing world.

As the pace of medical change increases, and as electronic communications and intelligence are deployed to an ever-greater degree in the provision of care, we will have the opportunity to reengineer the ways that we practice and consume medical care. The "ownership" of the medical record will move from the provider to the patient, so each of us will have more information about our own health and ways to improve it. We will have more information about which medical practices work best and how providers, be they facilities or individuals, perform relative to their peers. Medicine will change as radically and rapidly as other industries have. In the process of that transformation, we will have the opportunity to make medical care smarter and more efficient. Our challenge will be to create new models, like the patient-centered medical home, that integrate the promises of modern technology with the fundamentally human relationship that has evolved between patient and doctor in the thousands of years since Hippocrates practiced medicine in 400 BCE.

NOTES

CHAPTER 1   BED NINE DID DIE

1. "Neighbors Say They Knew Little About Pardus, Except For Concern For Mother," *Baltimore Sun*, September 17, 2010, http://articles.baltimoresun.com/2010-09-17/news/bs-md-pardus-neighborhood-arlington-320100917_1_mother-neighbors-south-kenmore.

CHAPTER 2   BONES

1. "Physician Smartphone Adoption Rate to Reach 81% in 2012, " Manhattan Research, October 5, 2009, http://www.manhattanresearch.com/newsroom/Press_Releases/physician-smartphones-2012.aspx.
2. Mike Rodewald, "UCLA engineer's telemedicine invention poised to begin trials in Africa," UCLA Newsroom, June 29, 2010, http://newsroom.ucla.edu/portal/ucla/ucla-engineer-s-telemedicine-invention-160653.aspx.
3. Leslie Tamura, "Physicians use photos from patients' cellphones to deliver 'mobile health,'" *Washington Post*, August 31, 2010, http://www.washingtonpost.com/wp-dyn/content/article/2010/08/30/AR2010083003939_2.html?hpid=sec-health.
4. Brian T. Horowitz, "Fujitsu Phone Lets Users Collect, Share Health Care Records," *Health Care IT News*, October 7, 2010, http://www.eweek.com/c/a/Health-Care-IT/Fujitsu-Phone-Lets-Users-Collect-Share-Health-Care-Records-474640/.

CHAPTER 3   SEE YA, IN 2015

1. "All quotes in this chapter are transcribed from a video John Pryor made on June 16, 1999 (http://www.drjohnpryor.com/John_Pryor/Biography.html)
2. Peter M. Warren, "For New Medical Students, White Coats Are a Warmup," *Los Angeles Times*, October 18, 1999, http://articles.latimes.com/print/1999/oct/18/local/me-23619.
3. Peter Warren, "For New Medical Students, White Coats Are a Warmup," *Los Angeles Times*, October 19, 1999, http://articles.latimes.com/1999/oct/18/local/me-23619/2.
4. The Arnold P. Gold Foundation, "History: The Power of an Idea," http://humanism-in-medicine.org/intros/gHistory.html.
5. "About Us," Arnold P. Gold Foundation website, http://www.humanism-in-medicine.org/index.php/aboutus/history.
6. "Doctors Recommend Smoking Camels," http://www.old-time.com/commercials/1940%27s/More%20Doctors%20Smoke%20Camels.html.
7. Prepared by Gilda S. Mann, Susan Stefanski, James M. Duffin, and Theresa R. Snyder, "I. S. Ravdin, 1894–1972, Papers, 1912–1972," University of Pennsylvania Archives and Records Center, Archival Collections, http://www.archives.upenn.edu/faids/upt/upt50/ravdinis.html.
8. "Welcoming the Class of 2014—from Vice Dean Gail Morrison, M'71, FEL'76," Penn Medicine Alumni August 2010 E-News, http://alumni.med.upenn.edu/august10news.php.
9. "Obituary, Dr. John Pryor," Philly.com, http://www.legacy.com/obituaries/philly/obituary.aspx?n=john-j-pryor&pid=121867510.

CHAPTER 4   CODE!

1. Stanford School of Medicine, eStudent, http://med.stanford.edu/estudent/.
2. "Will iPad Transform Med School?" PadTip.com: Apple iPad News, Help, Reviews, & FAQ, http://www.padtip.com/2172-will-ipad-transform-med-school/.
3. Ruthann Richter, "Philanthropist Li Ka-shing helps dedicate Stanford's new medical education building," Stanford News, September 29, 2010, http://scopeblog.stanford.edu/archives/2010/09/li-ka-shing-visits.html.
4. Michelle Brandt, "Mercury News highlights sophistication of med school's learning center," Stanford News, September 30, 2010, http://scopeblog.stanford.edu/archives/2010/09/sophistication-of-new-med-school-building.html.
5. Nina Tjomsland and Peter Baskett, "The Resuscitation Greats: Asmund S. Laerdal," Resuscitation 53 (2002): 115–119, http://www.laerdal.info/binaries/ABITAYKR.pdf.
6. Laerdal, SimMan® 3G, http://www.laerdal.info/doc/35957031/SimMan-3G.html.
7. Brian T. Horowitz, "GE Tests Smart Patient Room to Monitor Patient Safety, Cut Medical Errors," Health Care IT News, September 16, 2010, http://www.eweek.com/c/a/Health-Care-IT/GE-Tests-Smart-Patient-Room-to-Monitor-Patient-Safety-Cut-Medical-Errors-866750/.

CHAPTER 5   STRETCH, FLOSS, DANCE AND MENTOR

1. Susan Frith, "Prognosis Botswana," The Pennsylvania Gazette, March/April 2007, http://www.upenn.edu/gazette/0307/feature1.html.
2. Mary Schmich, "Advice, Like Youth, Probably Just Wasted on the Young," Chicago Tribune, June 1, 1997, http://www.chicagotribune.com/news/columnists/chi-schmich-sunscreen-column,0,4054576.column.
3. Ibid.
4. All of the quotations from Dr. Gluckman in this chapter were transcribed from privately filmed video of the speech he made to the incoming University of Pennsylvania medical school class on August 13th, 2010 at the school's Annenberg Center (unless otherwise cited).
5. "The Real Sherlock Holmes? Who was the real life inspiration for Sir Arthur Conan Doyle's fictitious detective Sherlock Holmes?" http://www.sherlockandwatson.com/the%20real%20sherlock%20holmes.html.
6. Wikipedia contributors, "Joseph Bell," Wikipedia, The Free Encyclopedia, http://en.wikipedia.org/wiki/Joseph_Bell.
7. Wikipedia contributors, "Nuremberg Code," Wikipedia, The Free Encyclopedia, http://en.wikipedia.org/wiki/Nuremberg_Code.
8. Frith, "Prognosis Botswana," http://www.upenn.edu/gazette/0307/feature1_2.html.

CHAPTER 6   DEAD PRESIDENTS

1. "All quotes from Washington's illness, treatments and death in this chapter are from this source." http://www.eyewitnesstohistory.com/washington.htm.
2. "George Washington and Eighteenth Century Bloodletting," Geocities mirrored site (October 2009) from Powell Valley News, http://www.oocities.com/~landerparker/washington.html.
3. "The Death of George Washington, 1799," Eyewitness to History website, http://www.eyewitnesstohistory.com/washington.htm.
4. Penn Medicine, "In the Beginning: The Story of the Creation of the Nation's First Hospital," History of Pennsylvania Hospital, http://www.uphs.upenn.edu/paharc/features/creation.html.
5. Ibid.
6. A brochure describing Franklin's commitment to public service and philanthropy, http://www.ala.org/ala/aboutala/offices/ppo/programming/franklin/materials/Section_Three_Layout1.pdf. Penn Medicine, "The Cornerstone," http://www.uphs.upenn.edu/paharc/timeline/1751/tline3.html.
7. Penn Medicine, "In the Beginning: The Story of the Creation of the Nation's First Hospital," History of Pennsylvania Hospital, http://www.uphs.upenn.edu/paharc/features/creation.html.

8. Penn Medicine, "Dr. Thomas Bond," History of Pennsylvania Hospital, http://www.uphs.upenn.edu/paharc/features/tbond.html.

9. Abraham Flexner, "Medical Education in America: Rethinking the training of American doctors," *The Atlantic*, June 1910, http://www.theatlantic.com/magazine/archive/1969/12/medical-education-in-america/6088/.

10. "Edward Shippen," Find a Grave website, http://www.findagrave.com/cgi-bin/fg.cgi?page=gr&GRid=18313283.

11. "Penn Biographies: William Shippen, Jr. (1736–1808)," University of Pennsylvania Archives and Records Center, http://www.archives.upenn.edu/people/1700s/shippen_wm_jr.html.

12. "A Sketch of the Early History of Practical Anatomy. The Introductory Address to the Course of Lectures on Anatomy at the Philadelphia School of Anatomy. Tuesday October 6, 1874," (full-text), Internet Archive, http://www.archive.org/stream/sketchofearlyhis00keeniala/sketchofearlyhis00keeniala_djvu.txt.

13. *The Continent*, an illustrated weekly magazine, conducted by Albion W. Tourgée (Our Continent Publishing Company, 1883), Item notes: v. 3.

14. Wikipedia contributors, "University of Edinburgh Medical School," *Wikipedia, The Free Encyclopedia*, http://en.wikipedia.org/wiki/University_of_Edinburgh_Medical_School.

15. "William Shippen Jr. (1736-1808),"Penn Biographies, http://www.archives.upenn.edu/people/1700s/shippen_wm_jr.html.

16. "John Morgan," U.S. Army Medical Department, Office of Medical History, http://history.amedd.army.mil/surgeongenerals/J_Morgan.html.

17. Address before the Massachusetts Medical Society, May 30, 1860, *The Works of Oliver Wendell Holmes, Standard Library Edition*, vol. IX, *Medical Essays* (Boston: Houghton, Mifflin, and Company, 1892), pp. 202–203.

18. "Oliver Wendell Holmes Quotes," QuoteDB.com website, http://www.quotedb.com/quotes/1518.

19. Abraham Flexner, "Medical Education in America: Rethinking the training of American doctors," *The Atlantic*, June 1910, http://www.theatlantic.com/magazine/archive/1969/12/medical-education-in-america/6088/.

20. Mark Hiatt, "Around the continent in 180 days: The controversial journey of Abraham Flexner," *The Pharos*, Winter 1999, http://www.rienstraclinic.com/info/FlexnerPharos.pdf.

21. Ibid.

22. Abraham Flexner, "Medical Education in the United States and Canada, " Carnegie Foundation for Higher Education, 1910, http://www.carnegiefoundation.org/sites/default/files/elibrary/Carnegie_Flexner_Report.pdf.

23. Doctors of the World, Netherlands: Perspective, http://adsoftheworld.com/media/print/doctors_of_the_world_netherlands_perspective?size=_original.

24. "Income, Earnings, and Poverty Data From the 2006 American Community Survey," U.S. Census Bureau, August 2007, http://www.census.gov/prod/2007pubs/acs-08.pdf.

25. The Dartmouth Atlas of Healthcare, 1999.

26. "Oliver Wendell Holmes Quotes," QuoteWorld.com, http://www.quoteworld.org/quotes/12293.

CHAPTER 7   GO FORTH AND MULTIPLY

1. Joseph Turow, *Playing Doctor: Television, Storytelling and Medical Power* (Ann Arbor: University of Michigan Press, 2010).

2. Ibid.

3. Robert A. Chase, "Proliferation of Certification in Medical Specialties: Productive or Counterproductive," *New England Journal of Medicine* 294 (1976): 497–499.

4. American Board of Medical Specialties, "About ABMS Member Boards: Visionary Leadership. Energetic Commitment," http://www.abms.org/About_ABMS/member_boards.aspx.

5. Frederick C. Cordes and C. Wilbur Rucker, "History of the American Board of Ophthalmology," *Transactions of the American Ophthalmological Society*, vol. 59 (1961): 296–392. http://www.pubmedcentral.nih.gov/picrender.fcgi?artid=1316413&blobtype=pdf.

6. Dorion Sagan and Lynn Margulis, *Origins of Sex: Three Billion Years of Genetic Recombination* (New Haven, CT: Yale University Press, 1986).

7. "Pediatrics at the Delta," Archives of *Pediatrics & Adolescent Medicine* 102 (1961): 671–676.

8. Douglas H. Erwin, "Macroevolution: Seeds of Diversity," *Science* 308, no. 1126 (June 2005): 1752–1753.

9. J.D. Salazar et al., "Cardiothoracic Surgery Resident Education: Update on Resident Recruitment and Job Placement." *The Annals of Thoracic Surgery*, 2006;82:1160–5.

10. "Goldendoodle," *The Full Wiki* website, http://www.thefullwiki.org/goldendoodle.

11. B. Klintberg et al., "Fewer allergic respiratory disorders among farmers' children in a closed birth cohort from Sweden," *The European Respiratory Journal* 17 (2001): 1151–1157.

12. "Adaptive radiation: Reference," *The Full Wiki* website, http://www.thefullwiki.org/Adaptive_radiation.

13. Atul Gawande, "The Cost Conundrum," *The New Yorker*, June 1, 2009, http://www.newyorker.com/reporting/2009/06/01/090601fa_fact_gawande?currentPage=.

14. Ibid.

15. Richard M. J. Bohmer and Thomas H. Lee, MD, "The Shifting Mission of Health Care Delivery Organizations," *The New England Journal of Medicine*, August 6, 2009, http://www.nejm.org/doi/pdf/10.1056/NEJMp0903406.

CHAPTER 8   SUCH WASTE IS TRAGIC

1. All quotes in this chapter from Wachter and Goldman are from Robert M. Wachter, M.D. and Lee Goldman, M.D., "The Emerging Role of 'Hospitalists' in the American Health Care System," *New England Journal of Medicine* 335 (1996): 514–517.

2. Coulee Medical Center, "History," http://www.couleecommhosp.org/Sub.aspx?id=1772.

3. Rickey Hendricks, *A Model for National Health Care: The History of Kaiser Permanente* (New Brunswick, NJ: Rutgers University Press, 1993), 51.

4. Ibid, 59.

5. Ibid, 81.

6. Cecil C. Cutting, M.D., "History Of The Kaiser Permanente Medical Care Program: An Interview Conducted by Malca Chall, 1985 University of California Berkeley," Kaiser Permanente Medical Care Program Oral History Project (Regional Oral History Office University of California), The Bancroft Library Berkeley, California. Accessed from Internet Archive, http://www.archive.org/stream/kaiserpermanante00cuttrich/kaiserpermanante00cuttrich_djvu.txt.

7. Ibid, 54.

8. Henry Kaiser quote, http://www.great-quotes.com/quote/756677.

9. Tom Debley and Jon Stewart, *The Story of Dr. Sidney R. Garfield: The Visionary Who Turned Sick Care into Health Care* (Portland, Oregon: The Permanente Press, 2009).

10. Sidney R. Garfield, "The Delivery of Medical Care." *Scientific American*, 222, no. 4, April 1970, 15–23.

11. Debley and Stewart, ibid.

CHAPTER 9   FOR ONE GOOD NEW SUIT OF CLOTHES

1. Wikipedia contributors, "Libby Zion Law," *Wikipedia, The Free Encyclopedia*, http://en.wikipedia.org/wiki/Libby_Zion_law.

2. Ibid.

3. "Report of the Fourth Grand Jury for the April/May Term of 1986 Concerning the Care and Treatment of a Patient and the Supervision of Interns and Junior Residents at a Hospital in New York County," Supreme Court of the State of New York, County of New York, 1986, Part 50.

4. "Yale's surgery program faces loss of accreditation," American Medical Association *News In Brief*, June 10, 2002, http://www.ama-assn.org/amednews/2002/06/10/prbf0610.htm#06101.

5. Juice, "Yale surgery residency stripped," *Student Doctor Network Forums* (blog), http://forums.studentdoctor.net/archive/index.php/t-31518.html.

6. "This Indenture," University of Albany, History 316Z syllabus, http://www.albany.edu/history/history316/JamesFranklinIndenture.html.

7.   "Report: Resident Duty Hours: Enhancing Sleep, Supervision, and Safety," http://www.iom.edu/Reports/2008/Resident-Duty-Hours-Enhancing-Sleep-Supervision-and-Safety.aspx.

CHAPTER 10   BINOCULAR VISION

1.   *The Elementary School Journal* 39, no. 2 (1939): 436–448.

CHAPTER 12   DOCTORS IN FLIGHT

1.   American Telemedicine Association, "Telemedicine Defined," http://www.americantelemed.org/i4a/pages/index.cfm?pageid=3333.

CHAPTER 13   MEDICAL AVATARS

1.   "Healthcare Reform Came Too Late for Joaquin Rivera," Philly.com, December 1, 2009, http://www.philly.com/philly/blogs/attytood/Healthcare_reform_came_too_late_for_Joaquin_Rivera.html.
2.   Wikipedia contributors, "Dominique Jean Larrey," *Wikipedia, The Free Encyclopedia*, http://en.wikipedia.org/wiki/Dominique_Jean_Larrey.
3.   Ibid.
4.   Steve Lohr and John Markoff , "Computers Learn to Listen, and Some Talk Back." *The New York Times*, June, 24, 2010, http://www.nytimes.com/2010/06/25/science/25voice.html.
5.   "Resources for the General Reader," Microsoft Research, http://research.microsoft.com/en-us/um/people/horvitz/layreader.htm.
6.   Ibid.
7.   Cindy Crump et al., "Using Bayesian Networks and Rule-Based Trending to Predict Patient Status in the Intensive Care Unit," *AMIA Annual Symposium Proceedings*, 2009: 124–128. http://www.ncbi.nlm.nih.gov/pmc/articles/PMC2815467/.

CHAPTER 14   SURVIVAL OF THE FIT

1.   Emma Cook, "The Desire to Define Ourselves," *The Guardian*, March 9, 2007, http://www.guardian.co.uk/lifeandstyle/2009/mar/07/personality-types-character-testing.
2.   "The Story of Isabel Briggs Myers," Center for Applications of Psychological Types website, http://www.capt.org/mbti-assessment/isabel-myers.htm.
3.   N. A. Stillwell et al., "Myers-Briggs Type and Medical Specialty Choice: A New Look at an Old Question," *Teaching and Learning in Medicine* no. 12 (2000): 14–20.
4.   Christine Laine and Barbara J., "The Good (Gatekeeper), the Bad (Gatekeeper), and the Ugly (Situation)," *Journal of General Internal Medicine* 14, no. 5 (May 1999): 320–321.
5.   Jorge D. Salazar, Peter Ermis, Antonio Laudito, Richard Lee, Grayson H. Wheatley III, Sean Paul and John Calhoon, "Cardiothoracic Surgery Resident Education: Update on Resident Recruitment and Job Placement," *Annals of Thoracic Surgery* 82 (September 2006): 1160–1165.
6.   "Louis Pasteur," Wikiquote website, http://en.wikiquote.org/wiki/Louis_Pasteur.
7.   "Are Your Fee Schedules Fair?" docstoc website, http://www.docstoc.com/docs/38109519/Are-Your-Fee-Schedules-Fair.
8.   Doctor of Nurse Anesthesia Practice website, http://www.dnap.com/.
9.   "Discussion Paper, Doctor of Nurse Practice," American Academy of Nurse Practitioners, http://www.aanp.org/NR/rdonlyres/9DC9390F-145D-4768-995C-1C1FD12AC77C/0/AANPDNPDiscussionPaper.pdf.

CHAPTER 15   MOTHER'S DAY

1.   "Retail Health Clinics," The American Academy of Family Physicians (AAFP), http://www.aafp.org/online/en/home/policy/policies/r/retailhealth.html.

CHAPTER 16   OUT OF NETWORK

1. President Obama Press Conference on Approval of PCMH Demonstration Project, December 9, 2009.
2. "Joint Principles of the Patient-Centered Medical Home: Principles Call for Changes at the Physician Practice Level to Improve Outcomes," American College of Physicians, March 5, 2007, http://www.acponline.org/pressroom/pcmh.htm.
3. The Kate B. Reynolds Charitable Trust, "About KBR," http://www.kbr.org/history-legacy.cfm.
4. John Buntin, "Health Care Comes Home," *Governing*, February 28, 2009, http://www.governing.com/topics/health-human-services/Health-Care-Comes-Home.html.

INDEX